Changes to "Magne
Exemplary Professi

Page 1: Insert the words: "G.   ,e in "The Magnet® Model"

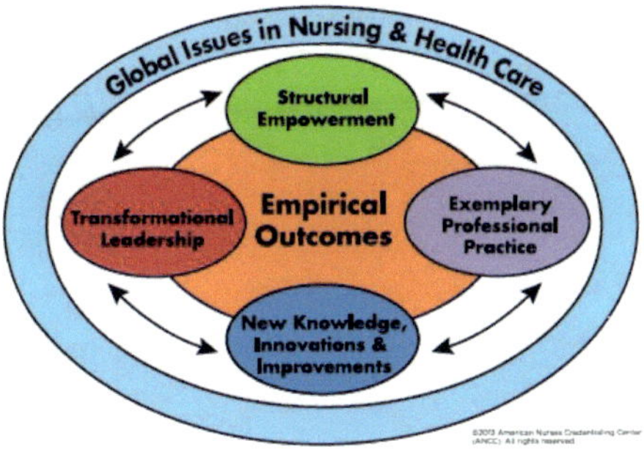

Page 20: Add the following text:
OO9
Provide the policy or equivalent evidence, which permits and encourages nurses to:
- Confidentially, express concerns regarding their professional practice environment, without retribution.
- Address the identification and management of problems related to incompetent, unsafe, or unprofessional practice or conduct.
- Address **interprofessional** conflict.

Page 23: Insert the phrase "in at least three of" is added to 6th bullet, so that it reads:
- The majority of the settings must outperform in at least three of the four registered nurse satisfaction/registered nurse engagement categories selected.

Page 47:
- All terms in the list of "Patient experience categories" should be bold and purple indicating that they are all defined in the Glossary.

Page 47 (continued):
- "f." should read "Patient engagement/patient-centered care" (slash added).

Correct list reads:

    a.   Care coordination
    b.   Careful listening
    c.   Courtesy and respect
    d.   Pain
    e.   Patient education
    f.   Patient engagement/patient-centered care
    g.   Responsiveness
    h.   Safety
    i.   Service recovery

MAGNET RECOGNITION PROGRAM®

EXEMPLARY PROFESSIONAL PRACTICE 2023

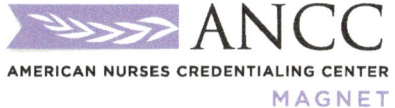

AMERICAN NURSES CREDENTIALING CENTER MAGNET RECOGNITION PROGRAM®

The American Nurses Credentialing Center (ANCC) provides people and organizations in the nursing profession with the tools they need on their journey to excellence. ANCC recognizes healthcare organizations for nursing excellence through the Magnet Recognition Program®. ANCC is the largest and most prestigious nurse-credentialing organization in the United States.

Magnet® Program Office

The ANCC's Magnet Program Office staff manages and coordinates all aspects of the application and appraisal process.

Contact information is available at nursingworld.org/organizational-programs/magnet/contact-magnet-staff/.

For Magnet Recognition Program information online, visit: nursingworld.org/organizational-programs/magnet/

For Magnet Application Manual Updates and FAQs, visit: nursingworld.org/organizational-programs/magnet/magnet-manual-updates-and-faqs/

American Nurses Credentialing Center
A subsidiary of the American Nurses Association Enterprise
8515 Georgia Avenue, Suite 400
Silver Spring, MD 20910
ISBN-13:
Print: 978-1-953985-33-0
Epub: 978-1-953985-35-4
ePDF: 978-1-953985-34-7
Mobi: 978-1-953985-36-1

Copyright © 2021 American Nurses Credentialing Center. All rights reserved. No part of this publication may be reproduced or transmitted in any form or by any means, electronic or mechanical, including photocopy, recording, or any information storage or retrieval system, without permission of the publisher. This publication may not be translated without written permission of ANCC. For inquiries or to report unauthorized use, visit https://www.nursingworld.org/organizational-programs/magnet/.

Disclaimers:

Please note this is an abridged version of the 2023 Magnet Recognition Program Application Manual. If your organization is considering pursuing ANCC Magnet Recognition®, the Magnet Application Manual is essential for understanding the full scope of application and documentation submission requirements. It is the only authorized publication that provides detailed information on the instructions and process for documentation submission.

Completing all the processes within the *Application Manual* facilitates Magnet recognition but does not, in and of itself, guarantee achievement.

Changes may be made by the ANCC to the Magnet Recognition Program and the *Application Manual* without notice. Applicants must confirm that they are using the most current edition of the *Application Manual* before preparing written documentation for submission to the ANCC Magnet Program Office. For application information and *Application Manual* updates, go to www.nursingworld.org/organizational-programs/magnet/.

The Magnet Recognition Program® Mission and Vision

Mission: The Magnet Recognition Program® will continually elevate patient care around the world in an environment where nurses, in collaboration with the interprofessional team, flourish by setting the standard for excellence through leadership, scientific discovery, and dissemination and implementation of new knowledge.

Vision: The Magnet Recognition Program will transform healthcare globally by bringing knowledge, skill, innovation, leadership, and compassion to every person, family, and community.

—*Commission on Magnet, 2020*

Contents

THE MAGNET RECOGNITION PROGRAM®
MISSION AND VISION   III

PREFACE   VII

CHAPTER 1   THE MAGNET® MODEL...................... 1

　　　　　　　Statistical Foundation: The Empirical Model   2

SECTION II   EMPIRICAL OUTCOMES (EO) COMPONENT ... 5

　　　　　　　Empirical Outcome (EO) SOE Examples:
　　　　　　　Presentation Requirements   6

SECTION V   EXEMPLARY PROFESSIONAL PRACTICE (EP)
　　　　　　　COMPONENT............................ 13

　　　　　　　Organizational Overview   18

　　　　　　　Exemplary Professional Practice   20

APPENDIX D   SOURCE OF EVIDENCE (SOE) EXAMPLES—
　　　　　　　TYPES AND WRITING GUIDANCE 57

　　　　　　　Empirical Outcome (EO) SOE Examples   58

　　　　　　　Source of Evidence (SOE) Examples Not Requiring
　　　　　　　Empirical Outcome (EO) Data [also referred to as
　　　　　　　a "non-Empirical SOE example"]   62

　　　　　　　GLOSSARY FOR EP COMPONENT   65

　　　　　　　REFERENCES   77

Preface

The American Nurses Credentialing Center (ANCC) and the Commission on Magnet (COM) are pleased to present the 2023 Magnet® Application Manual. This updated version (13th Edition) contains current information and instructions to guide Magnet® designated organizations as well as those considering the Journey to Magnet Excellence®.

ANCC Magnet designation is the highest credential a healthcare organization can achieve. It acknowledges the invaluable contributions of nurses in all healthcare settings and among all populations around the world. Magnet designation is an indication to **patients** and the public that these organizations have met the most stringent, evidence-based standards of nursing excellence in patient care delivery. It is a results-driven recognition that fosters nurse engagement, and the role nurses play as members of the interprofessional team to improve patient outcomes and reduce healthcare costs.

The revisions to the 2023 Magnet® Application Manual reflect evidence spanning 34 years of research and development. These revisions are driven by the improvements and progress seen in healthcare delivery systems around the world. The 2023 Manual was developed with input from subject matter experts including members of the Commission on Magnet, Magnet Program Office, and feedback from the field. Changes to the 2023 Manual clarify previous **standards**, acknowledge the importance of **diversity** of healthcare workers and patients, and expand upon standards in the context of an ever-evolving ambulatory care environment.

The Magnet Recognition Program's 2023 Mission and Vision inspire a sustained focus on patient care in interprofessional healthcare settings of excellence. The 2023 Magnet Application Manual standards continue to raise the bar for nursing with the ongoing development of new nursing knowledge and integration of evidence-based nursing practice. The value nurses bring to patient care, healthcare organizations, their communities, and the world is undeniable. Magnet designated organizations—of every size, patient-delivery setting, and in any location—examine and communicate a scientific impact on exemplary care delivery outcomes in the 21st century and beyond.

Jeanette Ives Erickson, DNP, RN, NEA-BC, FAAN
Chair, Commission on Magnet

Rebecca Graystone, MS, MBA, RN, NE-BC
Vice President, ANCC Magnet Recognition Program

Chapter 1

THE MAGNET® MODEL

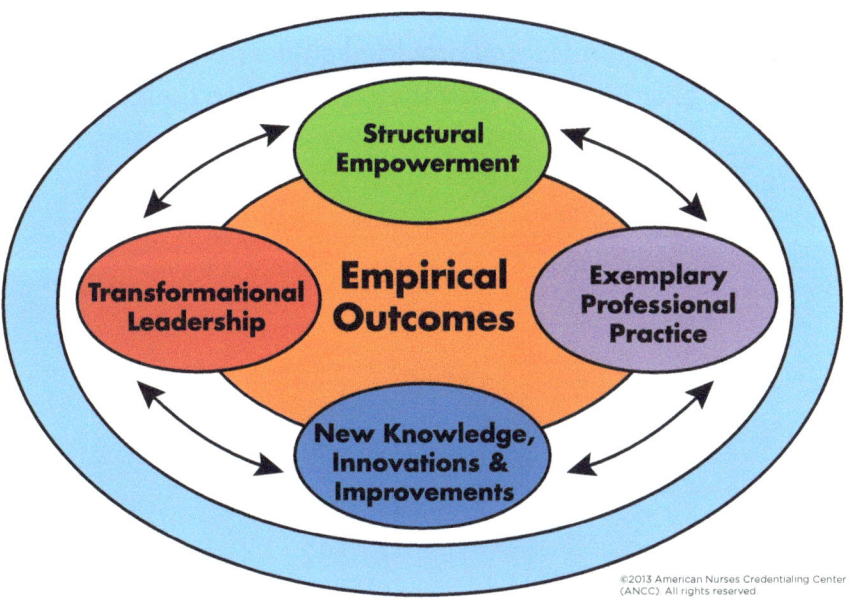

The Forces of Magnetism that were identified more than forty years ago have remained remarkably stable—a testament to their enduring value. The Magnet Recognition Program® evolved over time in response to **changes** in the healthcare environment.

Statistical Foundation: The Empirical Model

In 2007, the American Nurses Credentialing Center (ANCC) commissioned a statistical analysis of final appraisal scores for applicants under the *2005 Magnet Recognition Program Application Manual* (ANCC 2004). The project goal was to examine the relationships among the Forces of Magnetism by investigating alternative frameworks for structuring the Source of Evidence (SOE) examples and to inform development of the new Magnet Model. The newly developed Magnet Model first presented in the *2008 Magnet Recognition Program Application Manual* provided a new perspective on the SOE examples and how they combine to create a work environment that supports excellence in nursing (Figure 1.1).

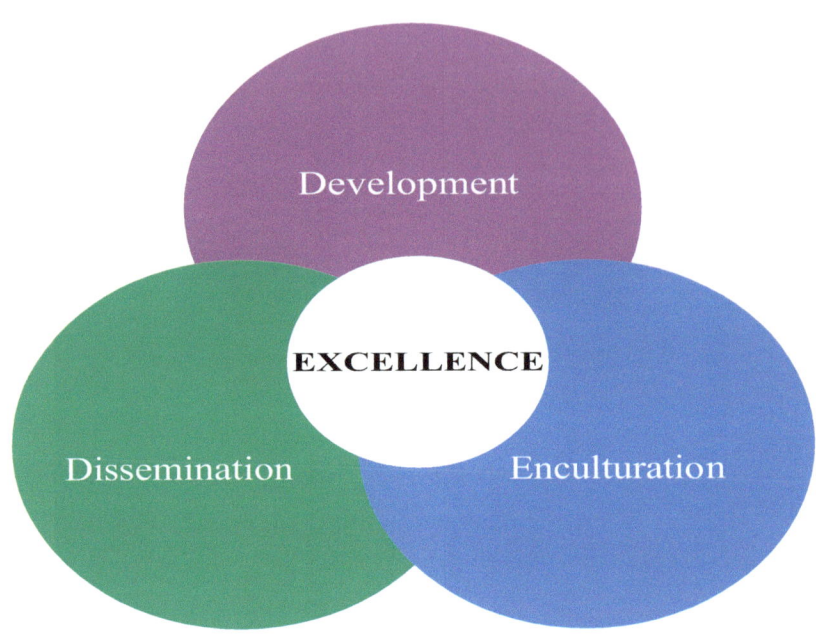

Figure 1.1. Triaxial Diagram

Through a combination of factor analysis, cluster analysis, and multidimensional scaling, the final SOE example scores were examined to determine how they might be organized based solely on their empirical properties. The results suggested an alternative framework for grouping the SOE examples. The empirical model yielded from this analysis informed the conceptual development of the current Magnet Model. Over the years, each subsequent manual has used a rigorous process, resulting in Magnet organizations creating a continued culture of excellence and innovation in nursing.

Excellence is determined through the evaluation of SOE examples, which demonstrate the infrastructure for excellence. The examples, provided by Magnet organizations, incorporate narratives to describe the structure and process used to achieve improved outcomes. These narratives demonstrate how the structures and processes are present and operationalized within the organization.

Before the *2019 Magnet Application Manual* was published, the Magnet Program Office (MPO) conducted an extensive evaluation of the characteristics of documentation submitted for review that met the threshold to move to the Site Visit Phase. The results indicated organizations that consistently demonstrated the development, dissemination, and enculturation of the Magnet Model Components in their documentation were the most successful. This finding established the expectation—for Initial Applicants and Magnet designated organizations alike—that the SOE example narratives and supporting evidence presented in an organization's documentation reflect enculturation of Magnet Component SOE requirements in their entirety across the depth and breadth of the organization, wherever nursing is practiced.

The 2023 Magnet Application Manual embraces the foundation set by the original study and ensuing Magnet manuals while acknowledging the importance of **diversity**, equity, inclusion and well-being of healthcare workers, patients, and communities; expands upon standards in the context of an ever-evolving ambulatory care environment; and raises the bar for nursing with the ongoing development of new nursing knowledge and the integration of evidence-based nursing practice.

Section II

EMPIRICAL OUTCOMES (EO) COMPONENT

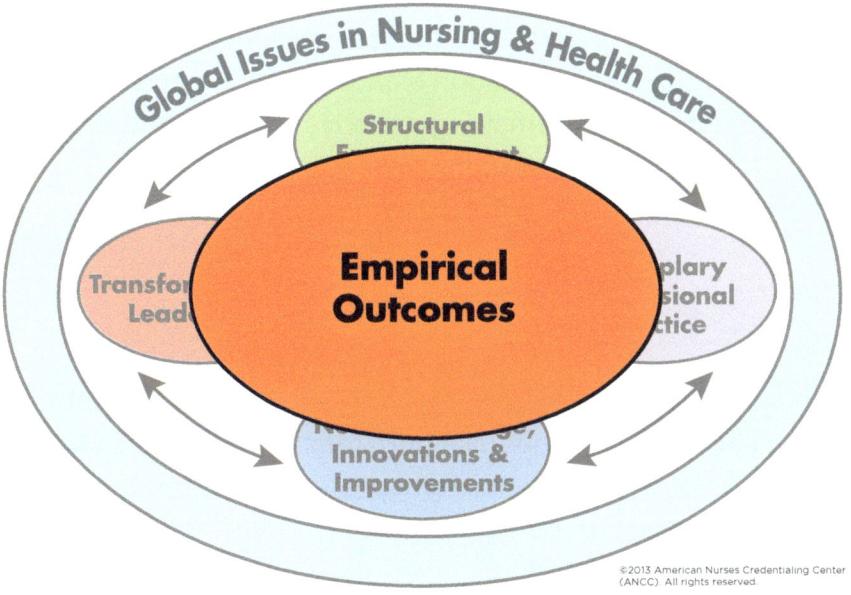

Professional nursing makes essential contributions to patient care, nursing workforce, organizational, healthcare, and consumer outcomes. The **empirical** measurement of quality **outcomes** related to nursing leadership and **clinical practice** in Magnet designated organizations is imperative. The 2008 introduction of the Magnet Model to incorporate outcomes represented a fundamental shift for the Magnet Recognition Program with the addition of the third component of Donabedian's Model of Quality—structure, process, and outcome. Previous Magnet Application Manuals emphasized **structure** and **process** and, although structure and process create the infrastructure for excellence in Magnet designated healthcare organizations, the impact of that infrastructure—outcomes—is essential to a culture of excellence and innovation. Outcomes demonstrate the achievement of desired results that are based on the healthcare team's application of sound structure and processes that exist within the organization and its systems of care.

Required Empirical Outcome (EO) Source of Evidence (SOE) examples are integrated throughout the Magnet Model Components in this Application Manual. Section II establishes the requirements for formatting narratives, graphs, and data tables, for the EO SOE examples.

Empirical Outcome (EO) SOE Examples: Presentation Requirements

Displaying data using graphs and data tables is an excellent way to illustrate outcomes resulting from the healthcare team's application of sound structure and process measures; therefore, a graph with corresponding data table (supporting evidence) is required for each EO SOE.

There are **unique EO SOE examples** that are identified in the bulleted list below that must be presented in specific formats. Specific presentation requirements for these unique examples are depicted within their respective EO SOE examples and located in the 2023 Magnet Application Manual on the page number(s) noted below.

- Page 40: Professional board certification (SE4EO)
- Page 41: Professional board certification (SE6EO)
- Page 45: Nursing education (SE8EO)
- Page 57: Registered nurse satisfaction/registered nurse engagement (EP3EO)
- Page 65: Nurse turnover rate (EP12EO)
- Page 69: Nurse-sensitive clinical quality indicators (EP19EO)
- Page 71: Nurse-sensitive clinical quality indicators (EP20EO)
- Page 74: Patient experience (EP21EO)
- Page 77: Patient experience (EP22EO)

All other EO SOE examples must be presented using the following Empirical Outcomes Presentation Requirements:

When using the empirical outcomes format, the example provided must have occurred within the 48 months prior to documentation submission.

PROBLEM

Describe the identified problem that exist(s) in the applicant organization that you worked to improve.

> **NOTE:*** The problem, pre-intervention(s), goal, intervention(s), and outcome *must* align.

> **Analysts' tip:** The outcome data drive the problem statement.

PRE-INTERVENTION

Describe the pre-intervention outcome data that drove the goal and initiative (must have occurred within the 48 months prior to documentation submission).

Describe the actions/activities that took place prior to the implementation of the intervention(s).

Include the timeline of dates of the actions/activities and the names of the key individual(s) involved.

GOAL STATEMENT

Provide the goal statement.

Include the outcome measure that aligns with the goal to demonstrate the improvement(s).

Include the location of the desired improvement.

> **Analysts' tip:** The stated goal *must* align with the graphed outcome data.

---

* *Information in NOTES is very important as it conveys a requirement and/or directive.*

PARTICIPANTS

- List participants involved in the pre-intervention and intervention activities or initiative.

- Include name, discipline, job title, and department.

INTERVENTION

- Describe the actions/activities that took place to facilitate the change and that had an impact on the problem to result in the achievement of the improvement/outcome.

- Include the timeline of dates of the actions/activities and the names of the key individual(s) involved.

- Include where and when the intervention(s) occurred (e.g., unit, department, service line, organization).

- Include a description of how the intervention(s) impacted the outcome.

- Provide key references (minimum of two) to support the interventions were evidence-based.

> **NOTE:** American Psychological Association (APA) format should be followed.

OUTCOME

- Provide **trended data** (i.e., a minimum of one pre-intervention data point and three post-intervention data points) demonstrating an improved trend.

- Pre-intervention and post-intervention data must be displayed to indicate the impact of an intervention or series of interventions on the outcome.

- The trended data must be displayed as a graph and table with data elements clearly provided.

> **NOTE:** The data point immediately prior to the intervention period cannot be zero.

> **Analysts' tip:** See glossary for the full definition of *outcome*.

DATA DISPLAY REQUIREMENTS

- The graph must include dates, location of data collection, legend, and title.

- Indicate on the graph the pre-intervention, intervention, and post-intervention timeframes.

- The *x*-axis units-of-time must be the same for pre-intervention and post-intervention data (e.g., quarters, months).

- The *y*-axis units of measure represent the desired outcome. Data must be presented as ratio (e.g., rates, percentiles, percentages). Additionally, the data must be consistent throughout the data collection period.

- If data are presented for a fiscal year, the period defining the fiscal year must be defined with calendar year equivalent (January to December and year; June to May and year).

- Pre-Intervention and Post-Intervention timelines must be consecutive and consistent (e.g., days to days, months to months, quarters to quarters, etc.) or time intervals that are consistent with established *performance improvement methodologies*.

- The Pre-Intervention, Intervention, and Post-Intervention periods may not intersect.

Analysts' tip: Align the timelines in the narrative and the improvements (outcomes) displayed on the graph.

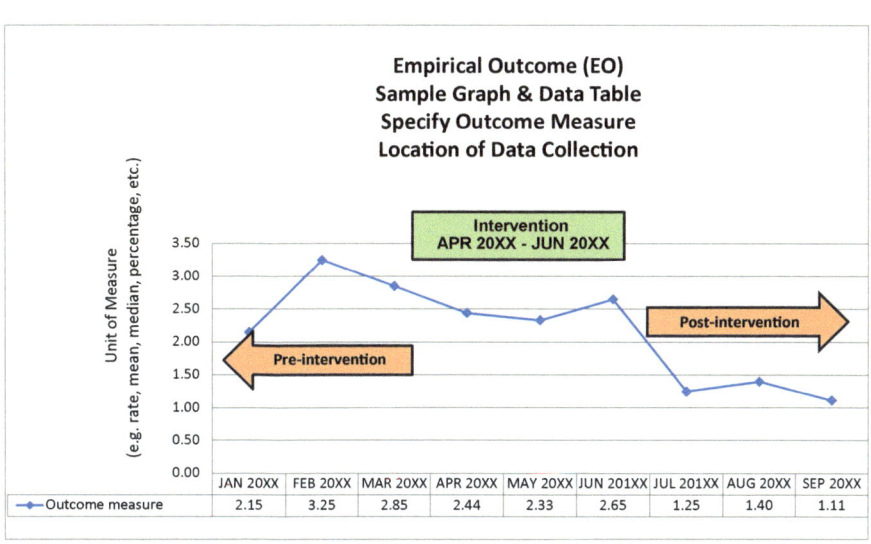

Figure II.1. Empirical Outcomes (EO) Sample Graph and Data Table

Section V

EXEMPLARY PROFESSIONAL PRACTICE (EP) COMPONENT

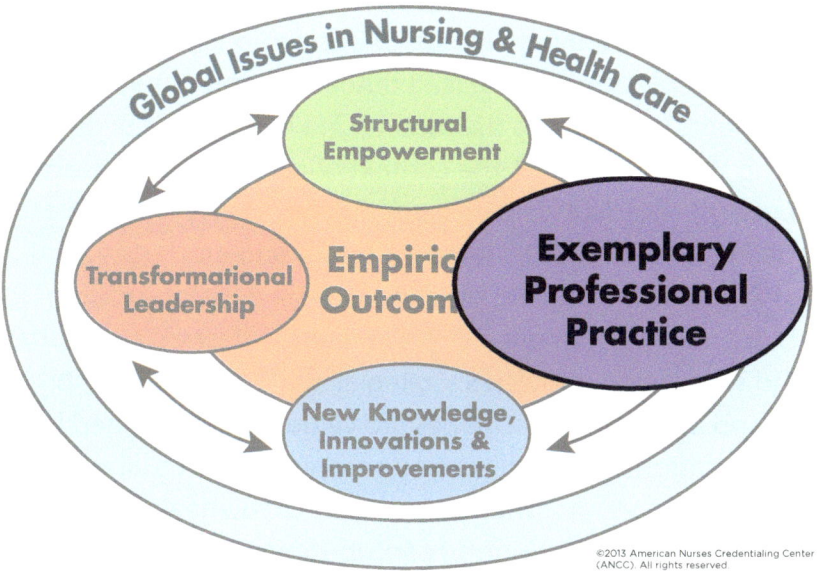

A **professional practice model (PPM)*** is the overarching conceptual framework for nurses, nursing care, and interprofessional patient care. It is a schematic description of a system, theory, or phenomenon that depicts how nurses practice, collaborate, communicate, and develop professionally to provide

---

* *This formatting indicates that these words and phrases are defined in the Glossary. Please refer to the Glossary for full explanations of these terms.*

the highest-quality care for those served by the organization (e.g., patients, families, and communities). The PPM illustrates the alignment and integration of nursing practice with the mission, vision, values, and philosophy that nursing has adopted. At the organizational level, nurse executives ensure that care is patient- and family-centered. Magnet® designated organizations take the lead in research efforts to create and test models that promote nurses' professional practice.

The healthcare delivery system is integrated within the PPM and promotes continuous, consistent, efficient, and accountable delivery of nursing care. The care delivery system is adapted to meet evidence-based practice standards, national patient safety goals, affordable and value-based outcomes, and regulatory requirements. It describes the manner in which care is delivered, the skill set required, the context of care, and the expected outcomes of care. Nurses create patient care delivery systems that delineate the nurses' shared authority and accountability for evidence-based nursing practice, clinical decision-making and outcomes, performance improvement initiatives, and staffing and scheduling processes. Collegial working relationships within and among the disciplines are valued and promoted by the organization's leadership and its employees. Mutual respect is based on the premise that all members of the healthcare team make essential and meaningful contributions to the achievement of clinical outcomes. Conflict management strategies are in place and are used effectively.

Exemplary professional practice in Magnet designated organizations is evidenced by effective and efficient care services, interprofessional collaboration, and high-quality patient outcomes. Magnet nurses partner with patients, families, support systems, and interprofessional teams to positively impact patient care and outcomes. Interprofessional team members include, but are not limited to, personnel from professions such as medical, pharmacy, nutrition, rehabilitation, social work, and psychology who collaborate to ensure the delivery of a comprehensive plan of care.

The achievement of exemplary professional practice is grounded in a culture of safety, quality monitoring, and **quality improvement**. Nurses collaborate with other disciplines to ensure that care is comprehensive, coordinated, and monitored for effectiveness through the quality improvement model. Nurses participate in safety initiatives that incorporate national best practices. Sufficient resources are available to respond to safety initiatives and quality improvements for patients and employees.

The autonomous nurse provides care based on the unique needs and attributes of the patient and their family, support system, or both. The knowledge, skills, and resources that have been identified by the nursing staff as necessary to practice are the foundation for the care delivery system; therefore, they are consistently available in the practice environment. Competency assessment and peer evaluation ensure that nurses deliver safe, ethical, and evidence-based nursing care.

Workplace advocacy initiatives include but are not limited to addressing ethical issues, patient rights, privacy, security, and patient and staff confidentiality. Magnet designated organizations embrace a culture that empowers nurses and other staff to identify and bring forth concerns without fear of retribution. Attention is given to achieving equity of care as well as equity in the Magnet designated organization's workplace environment.

Nurses at all levels analyze data and use national benchmarks to gain a comparative perspective about their performance and the care patients receive. Action plans are developed that lead to systematic improvements over time. Magnet organization data demonstrate outcome measures that generally outperform the benchmark statistic of the national database used in patient- and nurse-sensitive clinical quality indicators.

The intent of the Exemplary Professional Practice component is to reflect the following:

- Clinical nurses are involved in the development, implementation, and evaluation of the PPM.

- Nurse **autonomy** is supported and promoted through the organization's governance structure for shared decision-making.

- Unit- or clinic-level registered nurse satisfaction/registered nurse engagement data outperform the measure of central tendency of the national database used.

- Nurses collaborate with patients and families to establish goals and plans for delivery of patient-centered care.

- Nurses use **experts** to improve the clinical practice setting including clinician well-being.

- Nurses are involved in **interprofessional collaborative practice** within the care delivery system to ensure **care coordination** across the continuum of care.

- Nurses assume leadership roles in collaborative interprofessional activities to improve the quality of care.

- Nurses participate in interprofessional groups that implement and evaluate coordinated patient education activities.

- Nurses are involved in staffing and scheduling based on established guidelines, such as ANA's *Principles for Nurse Staffing, 3rd Edition* (2020), to ensure that RN assignments meet the needs of the **patient population**.

- Nurses collaborate during the budgeting process to distribute or redistribute nursing resources.

- Nurses participate in recruitment and retention assessment and planning activities.

- Nurses at all levels engage in periodic formal performance reviews that include a self-appraisal and peer feedback process for assurance of competence and continuous professional development.

- Nurses work within the full scope of their practice as defined by their **Nurse Practice Act**.

- Nurses use available resources to address ethical issues related to clinical practice.

- **Workplace safety for nurses** is evaluated and improved.

- Clinical nurses are involved in the review, action planning, and evaluation of patient safety data at the unit level.

- Nurses work with patients and families to improve patient experience.

- Nurses are involved in implementing and evaluating national or international patient safety goals.

- Unit- or clinic-level **nurse-sensitive clinical quality** indicator data outperform the measure of central tendency of the national database used.

- Unit- or clinic-level **patient experience** data (related to nursing care) outperform the measure of central tendency of the national database used.

Organizational Overview

The Organizational Overview (OO) items contain requests for documents and information that are foundational to Magnet® designated organizations and provide background information that informs the Magnet® Appraisers about the enculturation of the Magnet Components throughout the organization.

Exemplary Professional Practice

OO6

Provide a description and/or policies, or equivalent evidence of, the process by which the CNO (or designee) participates in the following:

- Credentialing, privileging, and evaluating of all **Advanced Practice Registered Nurses (APRNs)**.

- Reprivileging of all APRNs. Include the frequency of reprivileging.

> **NOTE:*** Designee *must* be a registered nurse.

OO7

Provide the policies, or equivalent evidence, that depict the organization's workplace advocacy initiatives for all staff, regarding the following issues:

- Caregiver **well-being**;

- **Diversity, equity,** and **inclusion**;

- Rights;

- Confidentiality;

- Care for the impaired practitioner; and

- Zero tolerance for **bullying**, **incivility**, and **workplace violence**.

> **Analysts' tip:** For more information, please refer to the American Nurses Association's position statement on *Incivility, Bullying, and Workplace Violence* located on the American Nurses Association's website. International organizations: for more information on this topic, please refer to the International Council of Nurses' statement on bullying, incivility, and workplace violence located on their website.

---

* *Information in NOTES is very important as it conveys a requirement and/or directive.*

Provide the policies, or equivalent evidence of, that depict the organization's initiatives for patients and families, regarding the following issues:

- **Diversity**, **equity**, and **inclusion**;

- **Cultural competence**.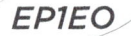

PROFESSIONAL PRACTICE MODEL

EP1EO

a. Using the required empirical outcomes (EO) presentation format, provide one example of an improved outcome associated with an evidence-based change made by clinical nurses in alignment with the organization's professional practice model (PPM).

- Provide a schematic of the PPM.

> **Analysts' tip:** Describe the alignment of the example to element(s) within your organization's PPM.

AND

b. Using the required empirical outcomes (EO) presentation format, provide one example, from an ambulatory care setting, of an improved outcome associated with an evidence-based change made by nurses in alignment with the organization's PPM.

▸ Provide a schematic of the PPM.

> **Analysts' tip:** Describe the alignment of the example to component(s) of your organization's PPM.

EP2

Provide one example, with supporting evidence, of clinical nurses using **shared decision-making** to change the nurse practice environment.

> **Analysts' tips:**
>
> ▸ Example can be from the unit, division, or organizational level.
>
> ▸ See the glossary for the definition of *shared decision-making*.

EP3EO

Provide all eligible **registered nurse satisfaction/registered nurse engagement** data to demonstrate **outperformance** of the benchmark provided by the **vendor**'s national database. Provide unit- or ambulatory care setting-level data for all settings (inpatient care, ambulatory care setting, and administrative settings) and include all registered nursing levels where collected and benchmarked by the vendor.

▸ Submit results of the most recent survey completed within the 30 months prior to document submission.

- Provide *overall* registered nurse participation rate.

- Select four of the seven **categories** listed below and present data for each setting. The four categories selected must be consistent across the organization.

  - **Adequacy of resources and staffing;** ✓
  - **Autonomy;**
  - **Fundamentals of quality nursing care;** ✓
  - **Interprofessional relationships** (includes all disciplines);
  - **Leadership access and responsiveness** (includes nursing administration or Chief Nursing Officer [CNO]);
  - **Professional development** (education, resources, etc.); and
  - **RN-to-RN teamwork and collaboration.** ✓

- Organizations that do not outperform on the *original* full registered nurse satisfaction/registered nurse engagement survey are able to submit results from a nationally benchmarked vendor **pulse survey** to demonstrate overall outperformance.

> **NOTE:** The *original* full survey would be the most recent completed full survey within the most recent 30 months prior to documentation submission. Provide the full completed survey in addition to the pulse survey for evaluation.

- ▸▸ The pulse survey must be administered after the original, full survey.

- ▸▸ Results from only one pulse survey must be presented. It must be the most recent pulse survey.

- ▸▸ For the pulse survey, the same four Magnet categories from the original survey must be used.

- ▸▸ Provide the overall registered nurse participation rate for the pulse survey.

- ▸▸ Overall outperformance rate will be calculated based on the cumulative results of the original, full survey and the results of the pulse survey for the selected settings.

▸ The majority of the settings must outperform the four registered nurse satisfaction/registered nurse engagement categories selected.

▸ To advance to Site Visit, registered nurse satisfaction/registered nurse engagement data must meet the scoring threshold for excellence in the Written Documentation Phase.

▸ Failure to demonstrate outperformance prior to Site Visit results in the conclusion of the appraisal process.

Analysts' tip: <u>International clients</u> refer to Appendix L and the Magnet Recognition Program website for more information.

Data presentation requirements:

- Display each unit or ambulatory care setting using the example provided on page 60 of the 2023 Magnet® Application Manual.

- There may be no more than two decimal places presented; in addition, there may be no rounding applied.

Categories

- Provide the four Magnet categories selected.

- The four categories selected must be consistent across the organization (inpatient, ambulatory care, and other settings).

- Refer to vendor to align survey questions with Magnet categories.

> **NOTE:** The vendor *must* provide a comparative measure of **central tendency** for the **category** as a whole, not for the individual questions that comprise the category. For Magnet purposes, the organization *must* provide their data for the category compared to the vendor supplied measure of central tendency.

Level of data

- Present data at the unit and/or ambulatory care setting level. If data are not available at the unit or ambulatory care setting level, present at the next aggregated level available from the vendor (e.g., grouped units, specialty clinics).

- Explain which units and/or settings are included within aggregated data.

- Explain which, if any, units and/or settings are not included.

> **NOTE:** The Unit Level Data Crosswalk™ (ULDC™) *must* display all units/settings where data are collected, and which units'/settings' data are aggregated by the vendor.

Benchmark

- Provide measure of central tendency from the vendor's national database.

- A different measure of central tendency may be used for each graph.

- Benchmark statistic must be depicted on the data table and *y*-axis of the graph.

Comparison group or cohort

- Provide an appropriate comparison group.

- Comparison group may change between units and/or settings.

- Comparison group label must be depicted on data table of the graph.

Graph presentation

▸ Graph(s) must include date (month, year) of the survey.

▸ Graphs may be presented using a single unit/setting or up to four units/settings on one graph.

▸ If two or more units/settings are displayed on one graph, the units/settings must use the same benchmark and comparison cohort.

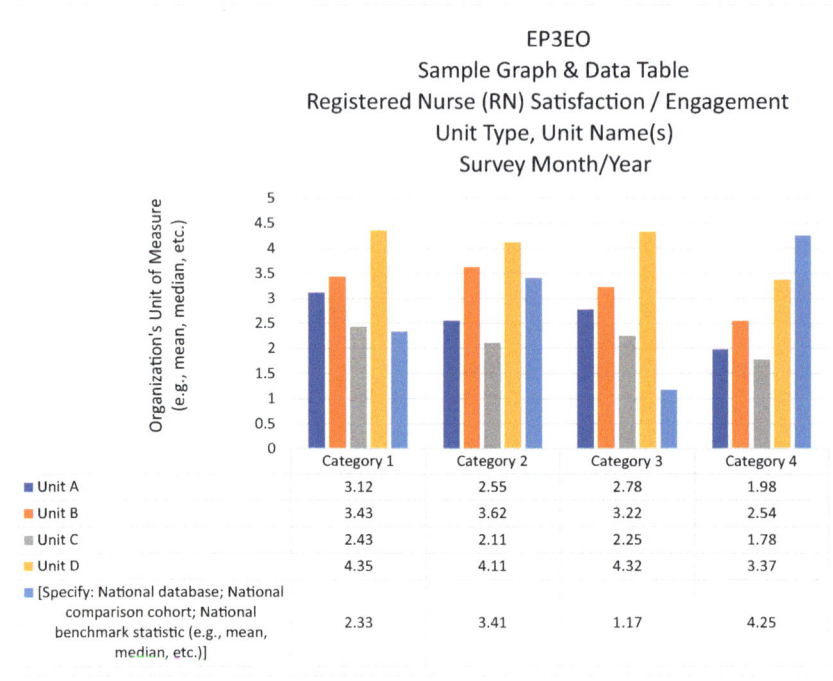

Figure V.1. EP3EO Example of Registered Nurse (RN) Satisfaction/Engagement Table and Graph

> **Analysts' tip:** If available, use vendor-provided graphs. Graphs *must* meet Magnet specifications.

Data presentation requirements for Registered Nurse Satisfaction/Registered Nurse Engagement Pulse Survey:

▸ Display each unit or ambulatory care setting using the example provided on page 60 of the *2023 Magnet® Application Manual*.

▸ Present results from only one pulse survey. It must be the most recent pulse survey.

▸ The organization must use the same four Magnet categories from the original, full survey for the pulse survey.

Categories

▸ Provide the specific category or categories selected for improvement in the pulse survey.

▸ Present pulse survey data only for categories which do not outperform on the full survey.

▸ Provide original, full survey data with the pulse survey data.

▸ Refer to vendor to align survey questions with Magnet categories.

> **NOTE:** For the pulse survey, the vendor *must* provide a national benchmark for the **Magnet category,** as a whole, not for the individual questions that comprise the category. All of the questions approved for inclusion in one of the seven categories specified *must* be included in the pulse survey.

Level of data

- Provide data for the specific units and/or settings selected for improvement in the pulse survey.

- Present data at the unit and/or ambulatory care setting level. If data are not available at the unit and/or setting level, present at the next aggregated level available from the vendor (e.g., specialty clinic groups).

- Explain which units and/or settings are included within aggregated data.

- Explain which, if any, units and/or settings are not included.

> **NOTE:** The Unit Level Data Crosswalk (ULDC) *must* display all units/settings where data are collected, and which units'/settings' data are aggregated by the vendor.

Benchmark

- Provide the measure of central tendency from the vendor's national database.

- A different measure of central tendency may be used for each graph.

- Benchmark must be depicted on data table and *y*-axis of the graph.

Comparison group or cohort

- Provide an appropriate comparison group.

- Comparison group may change between units and/or settings.

- Comparison group label must be depicted on data table of the graph.

Graph presentation

- Graph(s) must include date (month, year) of the pulse survey.

- Up to four units/settings may be presented on one graph.

- If the two or more units/settings are displayed on one graph, all units/settings must have the same benchmark and comparison cohort.

> **Analysts' tip:** If available, use vendor-provided graphs. Graphs *must* meet Magnet specifications.

EP3EO
Sample Graph & Table
Registered Nurse (RN) Satisfaction / Engagement Pulse Survey
Unit Type, Unit Name(s)
Pulse Survey Month/Year

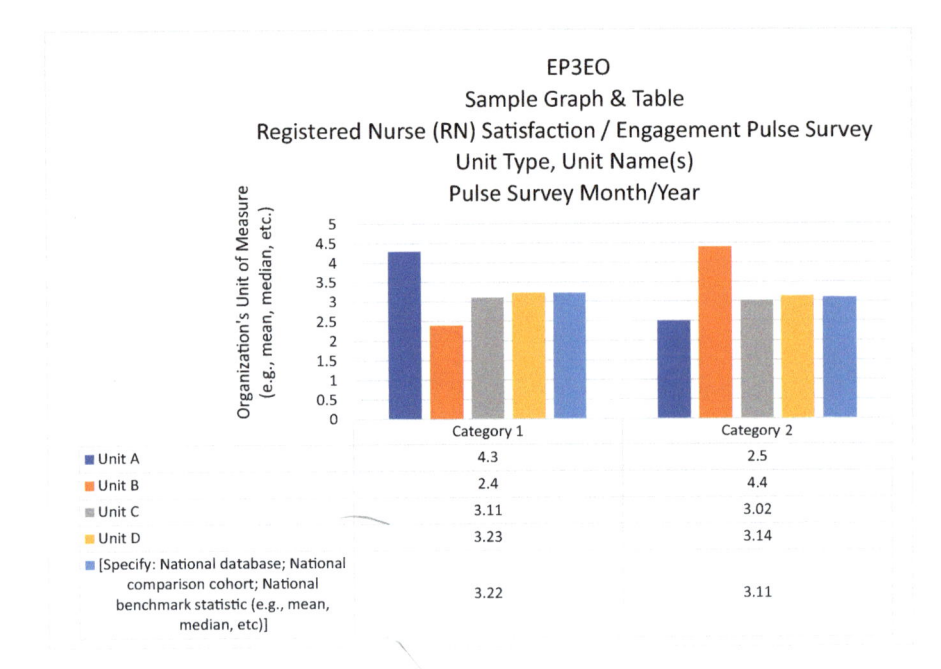

	Category 1	Category 2
Unit A	4.3	2.5
Unit B	2.4	4.4
Unit C	3.11	3.02
Unit D	3.23	3.14
[Specify: National database; National comparison cohort; National benchmark statistic (e.g., mean, median, etc)]	3.22	3.11

Figure V.2. EP3EO Example of Registered Nurse (RN) Satisfaction/Engagement Pulse Survey Table and Graph

CARE DELIVERY SYSTEM(S)

EP4

Provide one example, with supporting evidence, of nurse(s) **collaborating** with patient(s), families, or both, to influence change in the organization.

> **Analysts' tip:** See glossary for definition of *collaboration*.

EP5EO

Using the required empirical outcomes (EO) presentation format, provide one example of an improved patient outcome associated with one or more **experts**' recommended change in **nursing practice**.

INTERPROFESSIONAL CARE

EP6

Choose two of the following:

a. Provide one example, with supporting evidence, of nurse's(s') participation in interprofessional collaborative practice to ensure coordination of care from an inpatient setting to an ambulatory care setting.

b. Provide one example, with supporting evidence, of nurse's(s') participation in interprofessional collaborative practice to ensure coordination of care from an ambulatory care to an inpatient setting.

c. Provide one example, with supporting evidence, of nurse's(s') participation in interprofessional collaborative practice to ensure coordination among multiple ambulatory care settings.

EP7EO

Using the required empirical outcomes (EO) presentation format, provide one example of an improvement in a specific patient population outcome associated with nurse's(s') participation in an interprofessional collaborative plan of care.

EP8EO

a. Using the required empirical outcomes (EO) presentation format, provide one example of an improved outcome associated with an interprofessional quality initiative led or co-led by a nurse (exclusive of the CNO).

AND

b. Using the required empirical outcomes (EO) presentation format, provide one example from an ambulatory care setting of an improved outcome associated with an interprofessional quality initiative led or co-led by a nurse (exclusive of the CNO).

EP9EO

Using the required empirical outcomes (EO) presentation format, provide one example of an education activity led or co-led by a nurse(s) (exclusive of the CNO) for an interprofessional team which led to an improved patient outcome.

STAFFING, SCHEDULING, AND BUDGETING PROCESSES

EP10

a. Provide one example, with supporting evidence, when a clinical nurse(s) collaborated with a Nurse Assistant Vice President (AVP)/Nurse Director to evaluate data to address a unit-level staffing need.

> **Analysts' tip:** The unit-level staffing need may be related to a clinical nurse(s) and/or other types of unit staffing needs; however, the example *must* demonstrate a clinical nurse(s) collaborated with the Nurse AVP/Nurse Director to address the unit-level staffing need.

    AND

b. Provide one example, with supporting evidence, when a nurse(s) collaborated with the Nurse AVP/Nurse Director to evaluate data to meet an **operational need** (not work-force related).

EP11

Provide one example, with supporting evidence, when nurse(s) collaborated with a Nurse AVP/Nurse Director and/or Nurse Manager during budgeting to acquire new or redistribute existing resources.

> **Analysts' tip:** Budgeting refers to any point in the financial decision-making process. The resource acquired/redistributed does not have to be a part of a formal budgeting process.

EP12EO

Provide one example, with supporting evidence, of the organization meeting a targeted goal at the organization level, for improvement in the nurse turnover rate associated with clinical nurses' participation in nursing retention activities.

▸ Applicant organizations may use a maintenance goal if the organization nurse turnover rate is < 10%.

> **NOTE:**
> ▸ The example *must* include narrative about the clinical nurses' participation in nursing retention activities.
> ▸ If there have been extenuating circumstances within the organization within the three years prior to written documentation submission, the organization can reestablish a goal and show progress toward the revised goal. If this has occurred, describe the circumstances which led to reestablishing the goal.

EP12EO
Sample Graph & Data Table
Organization's Nurse Turnover Rate
Targeted Goal for Improvement

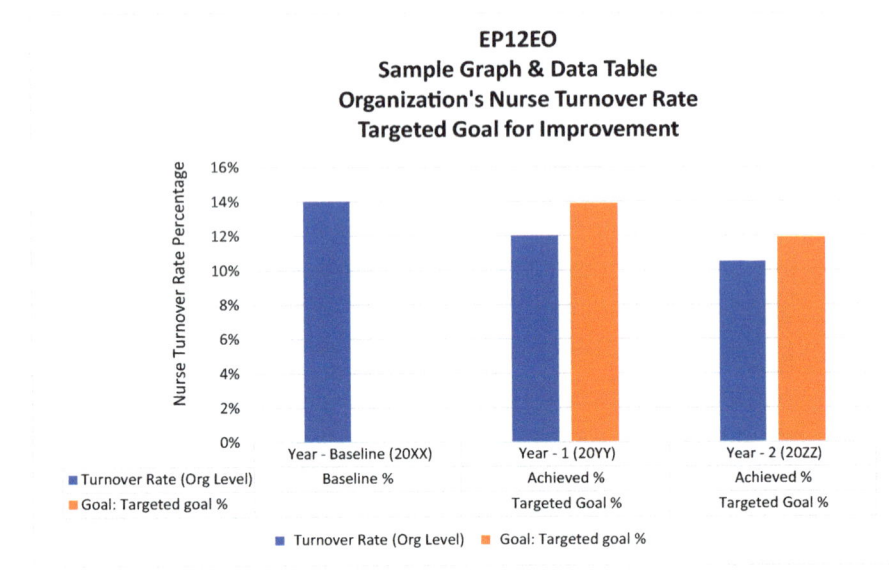

	Year - Baseline (20XX)	Year - 1 (20YY)	Year - 2 (20ZZ)
Turnover Rate (Org Level)	Baseline % 14%	Achieved % 12%	Achieved % ~11%
Goal: Targeted goal %		Targeted Goal % 14%	Targeted Goal % 12%

Figure V.3. Organization-Level (EP12EO) Nurse Turnover Rate

EP12EO
Sample Graph & Data Table
Organization's Nurse Turnover Rate
Maintenance Goal

Maintenance goal may only be used if an organization has reached < 10%

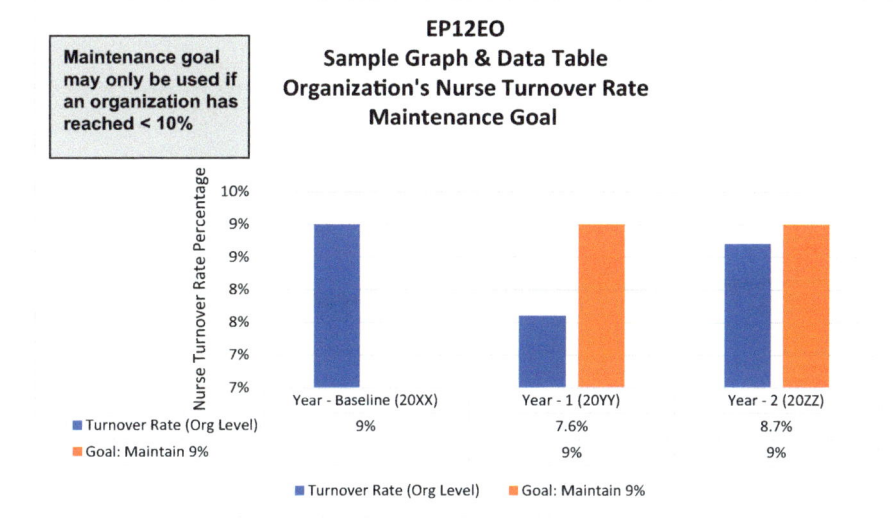

	Year - Baseline (20XX)	Year - 1 (20YY)	Year - 2 (20ZZ)
Turnover Rate (Org Level)	9%	7.6%	8.7%
Goal: Maintain 9%		9%	9%

Figure V.4. Organization-Level (EP12EO) Nurse Turnover Rate Maintenance Goal

> **Analysts' tip:** The intent of this Source of Evidence (SOE) example includes an organizational-wide nurse turnover rate. Cohorts are not representative of the entire organization and are not accepted.

EP12EO: Organization's Nurse Turnover Rate Data Display Requirements

The table and graph in this section represent the required format for illustrating that:

1. The organization has met a targeted goal for improvement in nurse turnover rate associated with clinical nurses' participation in nursing retention activities.

A graph must be labeled with date and title.

- A stated goal (percentage) for improvement in nurse turnover rate.
- Provide three years of graphed data to demonstrate the goal was met or exceeded.
- The first year represents baseline data.

ACCOUNTABILITY, COMPETENCE, AND AUTONOMY

EP13

Choose three of the following (**one must be from ambulatory care setting, if applicable**):

a. Provide one example, with supporting evidence, of the use of periodic formal **performance review** that includes a self-appraisal, **peer feedback** process, and **professional development** goal(s) for a clinical nurse.

b. Provide one example, with supporting evidence, of the use of periodic formal performance review that includes a self-appraisal, peer feedback process, and professional development goal(s) for a nurse manager.

c. Provide one example, with supporting evidence, of the use of periodic formal performance review that includes a self-appraisal, peer feedback process, and professional development goal(s) for a nurse assistant vice president (AVP)/nurse director.

d. Provide one example, with supporting evidence, of the use of periodic formal performance review that includes a self-appraisal, peer feedback process, and professional development goal(s) for an advanced practice registered nurse (APRN).

e. Provide one example, with supporting evidence, of the use of periodic formal performance review that includes a self-appraisal, peer feedback process, and professional development goal(s) for the Chief Nursing Officer (CNO).

> **NOTE:** The CNO example cannot be used as the ambulatory care setting example.

EP14

Provide one example, with supporting evidence, of clinical nurses having the autonomy to make nursing care decisions within the full scope of their nursing practice.

ETHICS, PRIVACY, SECURITY, AND CONFIDENTIALITY

EP15

Provide one example, with supporting evidence, of nurse(s), as participant(s) of an interprofessional team, applying available resources to address ethical issues related to clinical practice.

EP16EO

Using the required empirical outcomes (EO) presentation format, provide one example of an improved **workplace safety** outcome for nurses, specific to violence (e.g., physical or psychological violence, threats of incivility) toward nurses in the workplace.

▸ Provide a copy of the organization's **safety strategy**.

> **NOTE:** Outcome data *must* be specific to registered nurses.

EP17EO

Using the required empirical outcomes (EO) presentation format, provide one example of an improved patient safety outcome associated with clinical nurse involvement in the evaluation of patient safety data at the unit level.

EP18

Provide one example, with supporting evidence, of an initiative led or co-led by a clinical nurse(s), to address **patient experience** based on feedback from patient(s) and/or families.

EP19EO

Provide four nurse-sensitive **clinical quality indicators** for all eligible inpatient units. Data provided must reflect eight of the most recent consecutive and complete quarters of inpatient, unit-level graphed data to demonstrate outperformance of the benchmark provided by the vendor's national database.

Required nurse-sensitive clinical quality indicators for all inpatient units include the following:

a. Falls with injury

b. Hospital-acquired pressure injuries (HAPI) stages 2 and above

Select two other nurse-sensitive clinical quality indicators from this list:

    c. Assaults by psychiatric patients (inpatient psychiatric only)

    d. Catheter-associated urinary tract infection (CAUTI)

    e. Central line-associated blood stream infection (CLABSI)

    f. Hospital-acquired *clostridium difficile* (CDIFF)

    g. Device-related HAPI

    h. Multi-drug resistant organism (MDRO)

    i. Peripheral intravenous infiltrations (PIV)

> **Analysts' tip:** International clients refer to Appendix L and the Magnet Recognition Program website for more information.

Data presentation requirements:

▶ Display all eligible inpatient unit(s) using example provided on page 70 of the *2023 Magnet® Application Manual*.

- Data must be the most recent eight complete, consecutive quarters of data available from the vendor.

- There may be no more than two decimal places presented; in addition, there may be no rounding applied.

Level of data

- Present data at the unit level. If data are not available at the unit level, present at the next aggregated level available from the vendor (e.g., grouped units).

- Explain which units are included within aggregated data.

- Explain which, if any, units are not included.

> **NOTE:** The Unit Level Data Crosswalk (ULDC) *must* display all units where data are collected and which units' data are aggregated by the vendor.

Benchmark

- Provide the measure of central tendency from the vendor's national database.

- A different measure of central tendency may be used for each graph.

- Benchmark must be depicted on data table and *y*-axis of the graph.

Comparison group or cohort

▸ Provide an appropriate comparison group.

▸ Comparison group may change between units.

▸ Comparison group label must be depicted on data table of the graph.

Graph presentation

▸ Graphs may be presented using a single unit or up to four units on one graph.

▸ If two or more units are displayed on one graph, the units must use the same benchmark and comparison cohort.

EP19EO
Sample Graph & Data Table
Specify Nurse-Sensitive Clinical Quality Indicator
Unit Type, Unit Name(s)

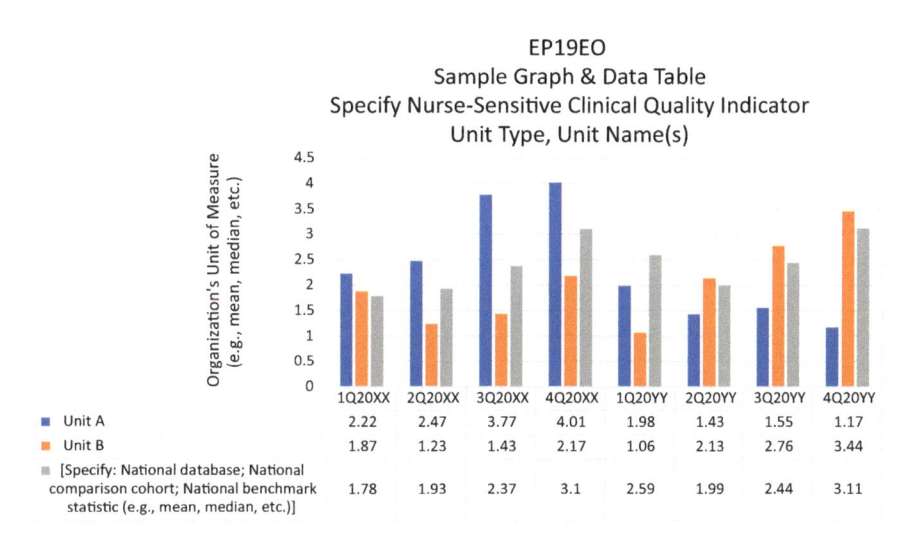

	1Q20XX	2Q20XX	3Q20XX	4Q20XX	1Q20YY	2Q20YY	3Q20YY	4Q20YY
Unit A	2.22	2.47	3.77	4.01	1.98	1.43	1.55	1.17
Unit B	1.87	1.23	1.43	2.17	1.06	2.13	2.76	3.44
[Specify: National database; National comparison cohort; National benchmark statistic (e.g., mean, median, etc.)]	1.78	1.93	2.37	3.1	2.59	1.99	2.44	3.11

Y-axis: Organization's Unit of Measure (e.g., mean, median, etc.)

Figure V.5. EP19EO Sample Nurse-Sensitive Clinical Quality Indicator Graph and Data Table

> **alysts' tip:** If available, use vendor-provided graphs. Graphs *must* meet Magnet specifications.

EP20EO

Provide *three* **nurse-sensitive clinical quality indicators** for all eligible ambulatory care settings. Data provided must reflect the most recent eight consecutive and complete quarters of ambulatory care setting graphed data to demonstrate outperformance of the benchmark provided by the vendor's national database or at the highest available level.

At least *two* of the ambulatory nurse-sensitive clinical quality indicators presented must be nationally benchmarked.

- Include a narrative describing how the selected nurse-sensitive clinical quality indicators are nurse sensitive in the organization.

- Include a narrative describing the benchmark used, including national benchmarks.

Suggested ambulatory care setting nurse-sensitive clinical quality indicators measures may include, but are not limited to:

- Advanced care planning;

- Ambulatory surgery hospital unplanned transfer/admission;

- Asthma care and follow-up;

- Body mass index (BMI) screening and follow-up;

- Cancer screening and follow-up;

- Comprehensive diabetes care: hemoglobin A1c (HbA1c) control;

- Depression screening and follow-up;

- Health literacy;

- Hypertension screening and follow-up;

- Multi-drug resistant organism;

- Patient burns;

- Patient falls with injury; and

- Surgical errors (e.g., wrong site, wrong side, wrong patient, wrong procedure, wrong implant).

For ambulatory-only organizations:

Provide *six* nurse-sensitive clinical quality indicators for all eligible ambulatory care settings. Data provided must reflect the most recent eight consecutive and complete quarters of ambulatory care setting graphed data to demonstrate outperformance of the benchmark provided by the vendor's national database or at the highest available level.

At least two of the ambulatory nurse-sensitive clinical quality indicators presented must be nationally benchmarked.

- Include narrative describing how the selected nurse-sensitive clinical indicators are nurse sensitive in the organization.

- Include narrative describing the benchmark used if there is no national benchmark.

> **NOTE:** This may include professional organization standard(s), literature-based, or an internal benchmark.

Data presentation requirements:

- Display all eligible ambulatory care setting(s) using example provided on page 74 of the *2023 Magnet® Application Manual*.

- Data must be the most recent eight complete, consecutive quarters of data available from the vendor.

- There may be no more than two decimal places presented; in addition, there may be no rounding applied.

Level of data

- Present data at the level of each ambulatory care setting(s). If data are not available at ambulatory care setting level, present at the next aggregated level available from the vendor (e.g., clinic groups).

- Explain which ambulatory care settings are included within aggregated data.

- Explain which, if any, ambulatory care settings are not included.

> **NOTE:** The Unit Level Data Crosswalk (ULDC) *must* display all ambulatory care settings where data are collected, and which settings' data are aggregated by the vendor.

Benchmark

- Provide measure of central tendency from the vendor's national database.

- Indicate the benchmark used if there is not a national benchmark available. A different measure of central tendency may be used for each graph.

- Benchmark must be depicted on data table and *y*-axis of the graph.

    - If benchmark is not provided quarterly, provide the reporting timeframe (e.g., monthly, annual) to include the equivalent of eight quarters of data.

Comparison group or cohort

- Provide an appropriate comparison group.

- Comparison group may change between ambulatory care setting(s).

- Comparison group label must be depicted on data table of the graph.

Graph presentation

- Graphs may be presented using a single ambulatory care setting or up to four settings on one graph.

▶ If two or more ambulatory care settings are displayed on one graph, the settings must use the same benchmark and comparison cohort.

> **Analysts' tip:** If available, use vendor-provided graphs. Graphs *must* meet Magnet specifications.

EP20EO
Sample Graph & Data Table
Specify Nurse-Sensitive Clinical Quality Indicator
Setting Type, Ambulatory Care Setting Name(s)

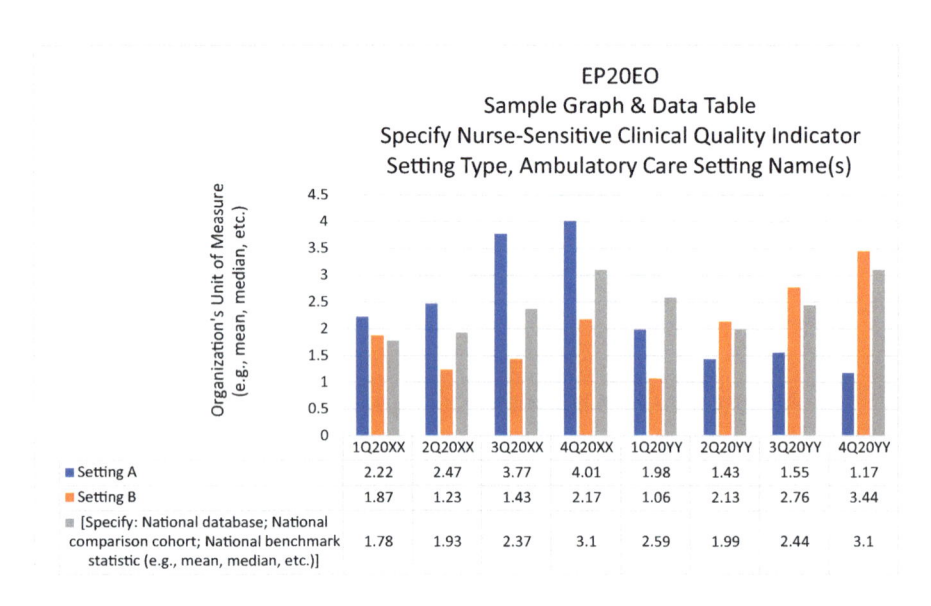

	1Q20XX	2Q20XX	3Q20XX	4Q20XX	1Q20YY	2Q20YY	3Q20YY	4Q20YY
Setting A	2.22	2.47	3.77	4.01	1.98	1.43	1.55	1.17
Setting B	1.87	1.23	1.43	2.17	1.06	2.13	2.76	3.44
[Specify: National database; National comparison cohort; National benchmark statistic (e.g., mean, median, etc.)]	1.78	1.93	2.37	3.1	2.59	1.99	2.44	3.1

Organization's Unit of Measure (e.g., mean, median, etc.)

Figure V.6. EP20EO Sample Nurse-Sensitive Clinical Quality Indicator Graph and Data Table

EP21EO

Provide four inpatient **patient experience** category data for all eligible inpatient units. Provide eight quarters of inpatient, unit-level data to demonstrate outperformance of the benchmark provided by the vendor's national database.

> **NOTE:** Data *must* be the most recent eight consecutive and complete quarters of data available from the vendor for all eligible inpatient care units.

Patient experience categories (select four of the following nine):

a. **Care coordination**

b. Careful listening

c. Courtesy and respect

d. Pain

e. Patient education

f. Patient engagement or patient-centered care

g. Responsiveness

h. Safety

i. **Service recovery**

> **NOTE:** Select *only* patient experience questions that the vendor has assigned to categories. Establish that the external vendor has collaborated with the Magnet Recognition Program® on alignment of questions to categories.

Data presentation requirements:

> **Analysts' tip:** <u>International clients</u> refer to Appendix L and the Magnet Recognition Program website for more information.

- Display all eligible inpatient unit(s) using example provided on page 77 of the *2023 Magnet® Application Manual*.

- Data must be the most recent eight complete, consecutive quarters of data available from the vendor.

- There may be no more than two decimal places presented; in addition, there may be no rounding applied.

Categories

- Present the four selected Magnet categories.

- Refer to vendor to align patient experience questions with Magnet categories.

- The four categories selected must be consistent across each of the inpatient settings.

- Within each Magnet category, the specific patient experience question may vary from unit to unit.

> **NOTE:** Select *only* patient experience questions that the vendor has assigned to Magnet categories. Establish that the external vendor has collaborated with the Magnet Recognition Program® on alignment of questions to Magnet categories.

Level of data

▸ Present data at the unit level. If data are not available at the unit level, present at the next aggregated level available from the vendor.

▸ Explain which units are included within aggregated data.

▸ Explain which, if any, units are not included.

> **NOTE:** The Unit Level Data Crosswalk (ULDC) *must* display all units where data are collected, and which units' data are aggregated by the vendor.

Benchmark

▸ Provide the measure of central tendency provided by the vendor's national database.

▸ A different measure of central tendency may be used for each graph.

▸ Benchmark must be depicted on data table and *y*-axis of the graph.

Comparison group or cohort

▸ Provide an appropriate comparison group.

▸ Comparison group may change between units.

▸ Comparison group label must be depicted on data table of the graph.

Graph presentation

▸ Each graph must include the Magnet category and the full text of the vendor-aligned question.

▸ Graphs may be presented using a single unit or up to four units on one graph.

▸ If two or more units are displayed on one graph, the units must use the same benchmark and comparison cohort.

> **Analysts' tip:** If available, use vendor-provided graphs. Graphs *must* meet Magnet specifications.

EP21EO
Sample Graph & Data Table
Patient Experience with Nursing
Specify Patient Experience Category
Include Entire Question Used for Categroy
Unit Type, Unit Name(s)

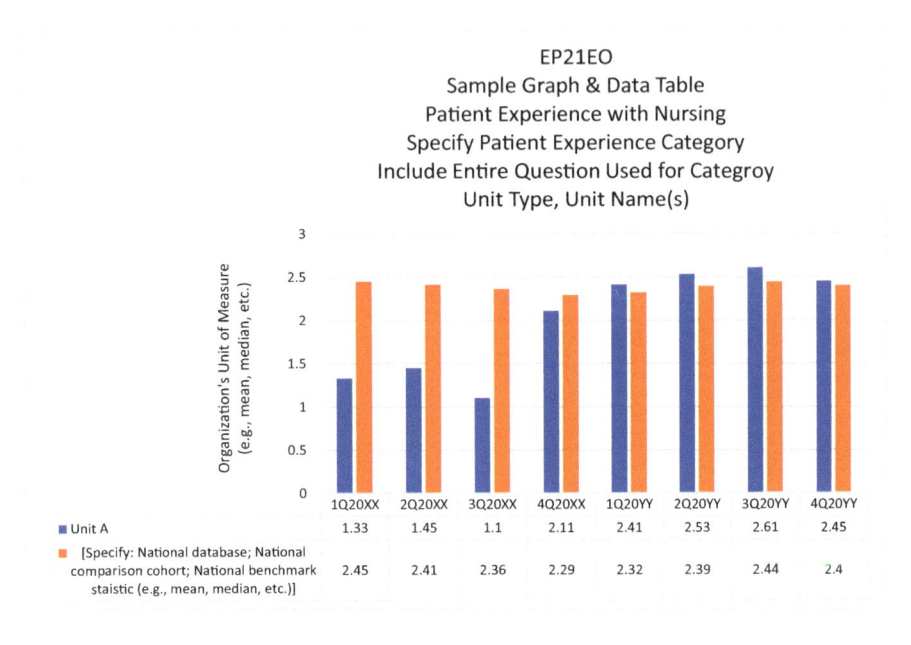

	1Q20XX	2Q20XX	3Q20XX	4Q20XX	1Q20YY	2Q20YY	3Q20YY	4Q20YY
Unit A	1.33	1.45	1.1	2.11	2.41	2.53	2.61	2.45
[Specify: National database; National comparison cohort; National benchmark staistic (e.g., mean, median, etc.)]	2.45	2.41	2.36	2.29	2.32	2.39	2.44	2.4

Y-axis: Organization's Unit of Measure (e.g., mean, median, etc.)

Figure V.7. EP21EO Sample Patient Experience with Nursing Graph and Data Table

50 | EXEMPLARY PROFESSIONAL PRACTICE 2023

EP22EO

Provide four ambulatory care setting patient experience category data for all eligible areas. Provide eight quarters of ambulatory care setting-level data to demonstrate outperformance of the benchmark provided by the vendor's national database.

> **NOTE:** Data *must* be the most recent eight consecutive and complete quarters of data available from the vendor for all eligible ambulatory care settings.

Patient experience categories (select four of the following nine):

a. Care coordination

b. Careful listening

c. Courtesy and respect

d. Pain

e. Patient education

f. Patient engagement or patient-centered care

g. Responsiveness

h. Safety

i. Service recovery

> **NOTE:** Select *only* patient experience questions that the vendor has assigned to categories. Establish that the external vendor has collaborated with the Magnet Recognition Program® on alignment of questions to categories.

Data must be included for the following ambulatory care settings:

- Emergency Department(s);

- Ambulatory Surgery Center(s); and

- All areas where clinical nurses provide care.

> **Analysts' tip:**
> - See glossary for the definition of ambulatory care setting.
>
> - Ambulatory-only organizations with non-traditional reporting timeframes, please refer to Appendix D.

Data presentation requirements:

- Display all eligible ambulatory care settings using example provided on page 80 of the *2023 Magnet® Application Manual*.

- Data must be the most recent eight complete, consecutive quarters of data available from the vendor.

> **Analysts' tip:** International clients refer to Appendix L and the Magnet Recognition Program website for more information.

- There may be no more than two decimal places presented; in addition, there may be no rounding applied.

▸ Data must be included for the following ambulatory care settings:

- Emergency Department(s);
- Ambulatory Surgery Center(s); and
- All areas where nurses provide care.

Categories

▸ Present the four selected Magnet categories.

▸ Refer to the vendor to align patient experience questions with Magnet categories.

▸ The four categories selected must be consistent across each of the ambulatory care settings.

- Different patient experience categories can be used for the ambulatory care settings compared to the categories used for inpatient.

▸ Within each Magnet category, the specific patient experience question may vary from setting to setting.

> **NOTE:** Select *only* patient experience questions that the vendor has assigned to Magnet categories. Establish that the external vendor has collaborated with the Magnet Recognition Program® on alignment of questions to Magnet categories.

Level of data

- Present data at the ambulatory care setting level. If data are not available at the ambulatory care setting level, present at the next aggregated level available from the vendor (e.g., clinic groups).

- Explain which ambulatory care settings are included within aggregated data.

- Explain which, if any, ambulatory care settings are not included.

> **NOTE:** The Unit Level Data Crosswalk (ULDC) *must* display all ambulatory care settings where data are collected, and which settings' data are aggregated by the vendor.

Benchmark

- Provide a measure of central tendency provided by the vendor's national database.

- A different measure of central tendency may be used for each graph.

- Benchmark must be depicted on data table and *y*-axis of the graph.

Comparison group or cohort

- Provide an appropriate comparison group.

- Comparison group may change between settings.

- Comparison group label must be depicted on data table of the graph.

Graph presentation

▸ Each graph must include the Magnet category and the full text of the vendor-aligned question.

▸ Graphs may be presented using a single setting or up to four settings on one graph.

▸ If two or more settings are displayed on one graph, the settings must use the same benchmark and comparison cohort.

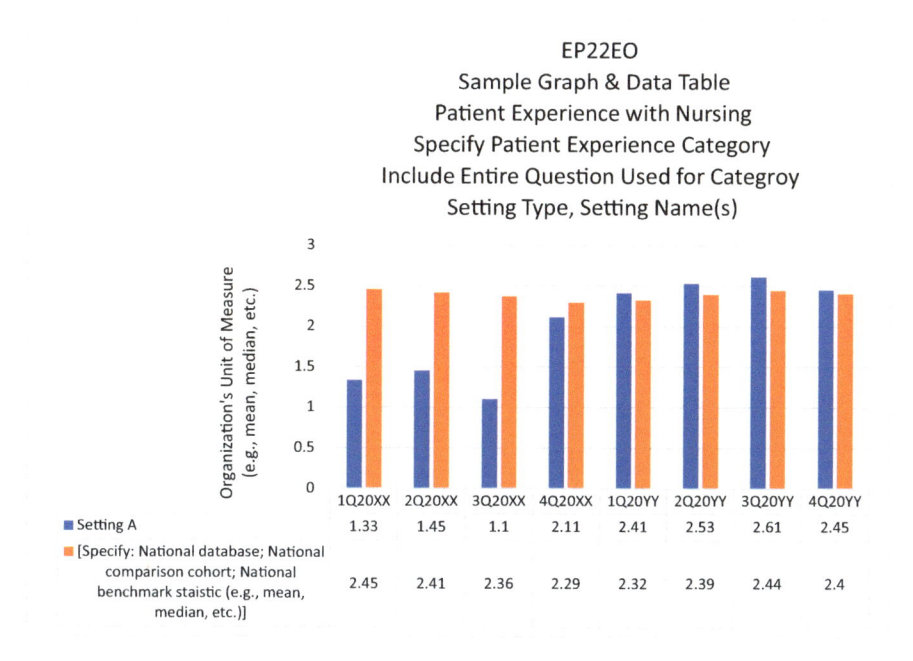

EP22EO
Sample Graph & Data Table
Patient Experience with Nursing
Specify Patient Experience Category
Include Entire Question Used for Categroy
Setting Type, Setting Name(s)

	1Q20XX	2Q20XX	3Q20XX	4Q20XX	1Q20YY	2Q20YY	3Q20YY	4Q20YY
Setting A	1.33	1.45	1.1	2.11	2.41	2.53	2.61	2.45
[Specify: National database; National comparison cohort; National benchmark staistic (e.g., mean, median, etc.)]	2.45	2.41	2.36	2.29	2.32	2.39	2.44	2.4

Y-axis: Organization's Unit of Measure (e.g., mean, median, etc.)

Figure V.8. EP22EO Sample Patient Experience with Nursing Graph and Data Table

---

Analysts' tip: If available, use vendor-provided graphs. Graphs *must* meet Magnet specifications

---

SECTION V: EXEMPLARY PROFESSIONAL PRACTICE (EP) COMPONENT

Appendix D

SOURCE OF EVIDENCE (SOE) EXAMPLES—TYPES AND WRITING GUIDANCE

The *2023 Magnet® Application Manual* requirements are organized by Magnet Model Components, which require two general types of formatting and supporting evidence as depicted below. The Source of Evidence (SOE) examples provided in the documentation submitted by the organization should depict the Magnet characteristics embedded in and enculturated throughout the organization. Each SOE example must be clearly identified and requires a separate narrative. Descriptions of processes or programs must be accompanied by examples to illustrate how each is operationalized within the organization. The written documentation should provide examples from different departments or units to represent a variety of specialties and nursing leadership in the organization. The goal of the narratives is to clearly illustrate how the examples depict a dynamic and innovative focus on excellence as well as how they are integrated and enculturated across the organization.

Information offered for additional clarity and/or direction throughout the Magnet Application Manual is highlighted as follows:

> **Analysts' tip:** information provided to serve as guidance

> information that conveys a requirement and/or
> e

Empirical Outcome (EO) SOE Examples

The EO SOE example narrative and supporting evidence must include:

- Problem

  - The identified problem that exist(s) in the applicant organization.
  - The problem, pre-intervention(s), goal, intervention(s), and outcome must align.
  - The outcome data drive the problem statement.

- Pre-Intervention

  - The pre-intervention outcome data that drove the goal and initiative
  - The actions/activities that took place prior to the implementation of the intervention(s)
  - The timeline of dates of the actions/activities
  - The names of the individual(s) involved

- Goal statement

  - The outcome measure that aligns with the goal to demonstrate the improvement(s).

---

* *Information in NOTES is very important as it conveys a requirement and/or directive.*

- The location
- Alignment with the graphed outcome data

- Participants

  - List of participants involved in the pre-intervention and intervention activities or initiative.
  - Name, discipline, job title, and department.
  - A meeting sign-in sheet is not required in addition to the participant list in an EO SOE example.

- Intervention

  - Description of the actions/activities that took place to facilitate the change and that had an impact on the problem to result in the achievement of the improvement/outcome.
  - The timeline of dates of the actions/activities and the names of the key individual(s) involved.
  - Where and when the intervention(s) occurred (e.g., unit, department, product line, organization).
  - How the intervention(s) impacted the outcome.
  - Provide key references (minimum of two) to support the interventions were evidence-based. Note: Follow American Psychological Association (APA) format.

- Outcome

  - Trended data (i.e., a minimum of one pre-intervention data point and three post-intervention data points) demonstrating an improved trend.

- ▸▸ Pre-intervention and post-intervention data must be displayed to indicate the impact of an intervention or series of interventions on the outcome.

- ▸▸ The trended data must be displayed as a graph and table with data elements clearly provided.

▸ Data display requirements are also found in the 2023 Magnet Application Manual, Chapter 3, page 26.

> **IMPORTANT:** All examples and supporting evidence *must* have occurred within the 48 months prior to documentation submission. This requirement includes data presentation See Appendix C Timelines for exceptions to this requirement.

▸ The graphed outcome data, presented to substantiate the example narrative, represent the supporting evidence.

▸ Align the timelines in the narrative with the data displayed on the graph.

▸ Outcome data must be presented as a ratio (e.g., rate, percentage, average, mean, median) consistently throughout the data collection period. The only exception is with a "sentinel" or "never" event.

▸ A limited number of EO SOE examples require specific supporting documentation. This will be depicted in the example.

▸ Redact all protected health information (PHI).

Unique EO SOE Example presentations are required and depicted within the respective EO SOE examples in the 2023 Magnet Application Manual:

- Page 40: Professional board certification (SE4EO)

- Page 41: Professional board certification (SE6EO)

- Page 45: Nursing education (SE8EO)

- Page 57: Registered nurse satisfaction/registered nurse engagement (EP3EO)

- Page 65: Nurse turnover rate (EP12EO)

- Page 69: Nurse-sensitive clinical quality indicators (EP19EO)

- Page 71: Nurse-sensitive clinical quality indicators (EP20EO)

- Page 74: Patient engagement (EP21EO)

- Page 77: Patient engagement (EP22EO)

Inpatient vs. ambulatory setting examples:

- If two examples are requested (one ambulatory/one inpatient) and ambulatory settings do not exist in the organization, then two inpatient setting examples must be provided.

- If the EO SOE example request is not specific regarding the inpatient or ambulatory care setting, the example may be written about either setting.

- Ambulatory organizations that do not have any inpatient settings provide only ambulatory examples.

- Ambulatory examples must be specific to the ambulatory setting; all data must be from the ambulatory setting as well.

- Benchmarked data specific only to ambulatory units/areas: if a quarterly benchmark is not available, provide the available reporting timeframe (e.g., monthly, annual) to represent the equivalent of eight quarters of benchmarked data.

Source of Evidence (SOE) Examples Not Requiring Empirical Outcome (EO) Data [also referred to as a "Non-Empirical SOE example"]

The non-EO SOE examples and supporting evidence must occur within the 48-month period prior to the submission of written documentation. All protected health information (PHI) must be redacted before documentation submission.

The non-EO SOE example is written as follows:

- Narrative Statement: A description that concisely conveys how the key elements of the SOE example statement are present and operationalized within the organization. The Narrative Statement:

    - Must be a straightforward and concise description of how the SOE example is present and operationalized within the organization.

    - Must address the key words and phrases (key elements) in the SOE request statement.

    - Organizations with flat organizational structures, such as without Nurse Managers: the Nurse AVP/Nurse Director may be substituted for Nurse Manager SOE example(s).

- Example must have occurred within the 48 months prior to documentation submission.

> **IMPORTANT:** The use of the EO SOE example outline template should <u>not</u> be used when writing non-EO SOE examples.

- Supporting evidence:

    - Comprised of item(s) that support and substantiate what is stated in the narrative statements which must have occurred within the 48 months prior to documentation submission.
    - Verifies that what is stated in the narrative exists in the organization.
    - Must substantiate narrative that addresses the key words and phrases (key elements) in the SOE request statement.
    - Limit of five supporting evidence items per non-EO SOE example.
    - Acceptable supporting evidence includes (but is not limited to):
        - Copies of written policies and procedures, files, intranet sites, meeting minutes, various types of correspondence, data, rosters, committee charters, job descriptions, and screenshots.
    - To be valid, supporting evidence must:
        - Be dated;
        - Contain signatures (as applicable);
        - Be legible; and

- Include participants described in the example (e.g., name, position, title), as applicable.

▶▶ Supporting evidence does not include:

- Photographs;
- Testimonial statements; and
- Documents generated for the purpose of clarifying the narrative.

Inpatient vs. ambulatory setting examples:

▶ If the SOE example request is not specific regarding the inpatient or ambulatory care setting, the example may be written about either setting.

▶ If two examples are requested (one ambulatory/one inpatient) and the organization does not include ambulatory settings, then two inpatient setting examples must be provided. Ambulatory organizations that do not have any inpatient settings provide only ambulatory examples.

▶ SOE examples that request narrative specific to ambulatory areas must be specific to the ambulatory setting. The narrative cannot take place in both inpatient and ambulatory areas.

> **Analysts' tip:** The Magnet Program Office strongly recommends participation in the webinar Preparing a Successful Document—Critical Information. This webinar is available to applicants or members of the Magnet Learning Communities. Data indicate there is a corresponding increased success rate for organizations that view the webinar. For information, contact your regional **Magnet Program Specialist (MPS)**.

GLOSSARY FOR EP COMPONENT

accountability
"To be *answerable* to oneself and others for one's own choices, decisions, and actions as measured against a standard such as that established by the *Code of Ethics for Nurses with Interpretive Statements*" (American Nurses Association, 2015a, p. 41). "The primary goals of professional accountability in nursing are to maintain high standards of care and to protect the patient from harm. All nurses are accountable for the proper use of their knowledge and skills in the provision of care" (Farquharson, 2004, pp. 311–312).

adequacy of resources and staffing
One of seven Magnet® optional categories for registered nurse satisfaction/registered nurse engagement. This survey category must include a minimum of two pre-approved questions that reference staffing and adequacy of resources.

advanced practice registered nurse (APRN)
"A subset of graduate-level prepared registered nurses who have completed an accredited graduate-level education program preparing the nurse for special licensure and practice for one of the four recognized APRN roles: certified registered nurse anesthetist (CRNA), certified nurse-midwife (CNM), clinical nurse specialist (CNS), or certified nurse practitioner (CNP)" (American Nurses Association, 2021).

autonomy
Aspects of autonomy include:

- Control over nursing practice: Refers to the authority and freedom of nurses to engage in nursing practice decision-making (within the full scope of their practice) that includes organizational structures, governance, rules, policies, and operations (adapted from Weston, 2010).

- Clinical autonomy: Refers to authority and freedom of nurses to make nursing care decisions (within the full scope of their practice) in the clinical care of patients within interprofessional practice environments (adapted from Weston, 2010).

- Organizational autonomy: Refers to the authority and the freedom of a nurse to be involved in broader unit, service line, organization, or system decision-making processes pertaining to patient care, policies and procedures, and work environment (adapted from Weston, 2010).

Additionally, one of seven optional Magnet® categories for registered nurse satisfaction/registered nurse engagement. Each of the aspects of autonomy must be covered in this survey category.

bullying
Bullying is repeated, unwanted harmful actions intended to humiliate, offend, and cause distress in the recipient. Bullying actions include those that harm, undermine, and degrade. Actions may include, but are not limited to, hostile remarks, verbal attacks, threats, taunts, intimidation, and withholding of support (American Nurses Association, 2015a).

care coordination
One of nine optional Magnet categories for patient experience.

"Care coordination is the deliberate organization of patient care activities between two or more participants (including the patient) involved in the patient's care to facilitate the appropriate delivery of health care services" (Agency for Healthcare Research and Quality, 2014, June).

category

See *Magnet® category*.

central tendency

An index that comes from the center of a distribution of scores, describing what is a "typical" value; the most common indices of central tendency are the mode, median and the mean (Polit, 2010, p. 398).

clinical practice

For Magnet purposes, refers to the care of patients provided in a healthcare setting.

clinical quality indicators

Clinical quality indicators are standardized, evidence-based measures of healthcare quality that can be used to measure and track clinical performance and outcomes (Agency for Healthcare Research and Quality, 2020).

collaboration

"Collaboration is both a process and an outcome in which shared interest or conflict that cannot be addressed by any single individual is addressed by key stakeholders. . . . The collaborative process involves a synthesis of different perspectives to better understand complex problems. A collaborative outcome is the development of integrative solutions that go beyond an individual vision to a productive resolution that could not be accomplished by any single person or organization" (Gardner, 2005, p. 1).

cultural competence
The integration and transformation of knowledge about individuals and groups of people into specific standards, policies, practices, and attitudes used in appropriate cultural settings to increase the quality of services; thereby producing better outcomes (National Prevention Information Network, 2020).

diversity
"The multiplicity of human differences among groups of people or individuals. Increasing diversity means enhancing one's ability to recognize, understand, and respect the differences that may exist between groups and individuals. Increasing diversity in the healthcare workforce requires recognition of many other dimensions, including, but not limited to gender, sexual orientation, race, ethnicity, nationality, religion, age, cultural background, socio-economic status, disabilities, and language" (National Advisory Council on Nurse Education and Practice, 2013). Fostering diversity involves building an atmosphere of inclusiveness.

equity
"Justice according to natural law or right; freedom from bias or favoritism" (Merriam-Webster, n.d.).

expert
A person "having, involving, or displaying special skill or knowledge deriving from training or experience" (Merriam-Webster, n.d.).

fundamentals of quality nursing care
One of seven optional Magnet categories for registered nurse satisfaction/registered nurse engagement benchmarking. Each

of the following fundamental aspects of quality nursing care must be covered in this survey category:

- The Nursing Professional Practice Model illustrates the alignment and integration of nursing integration of nursing practice with the mission, vision, philosophy, and values of the organization.

- Nursing leadership develops a strong vision and well-articulated philosophy that supports and promotes high standards for nursing practice.

- Nurses are clinically competent.

- Nurses incorporate evidence-based findings and standards findings and standards into the delivery of patient care.

- Nurses partner with patients and families to diagnose plan and deliver individualized patient-centered care.

- A culture of safety is promoted in the nurse work environment.

- Nurses participate in the surveillance, reporting, and evaluation of continuous quality improvement.

incivility

Incivility can take the form of rude and discourteous actions, of gossiping and spreading rumors, and of refusing to assist a coworker. All of those are an affront to the dignity of a coworker and violate professional standards of respect. Such actions may also include name-calling, using a condescending tone, and expressing public criticism (American Nurses Association, 2015a).

inclusion
"The act or practice of including and accommodating people who have historically been excluded (as because of their race, gender, sexuality, or ability)" (Merriam-Webster, n.d.).

interprofessional collaboration
"Occurs when healthcare professionals of diverse backgrounds and differing professional cultures work together to provide care that addresses a patient's needs" (D'Amour & Oandasan, 2005).

interprofessional collaborative practice
"Occurs when multiple health workers from different professional backgrounds provide comprehensive services by working with patients, their families, caregivers, and communities to deliver the highest quality of care across settings. Practice includes both clinical and non-clinical health-related work, such as diagnosis, treatment, surveillance, health communications, management and sanitation engineering" (World Health Organization, 2010, p. 13).

interprofessional relationships
One of seven optional Magnet categories for registered nurse satisfaction/ registered nurse engagement benchmarking. This survey category must include a minimum of two pre-approved questions that reference all disciplines.

leadership access and responsiveness
One of seven optional Magnet categories for registered nurse satisfaction/ registered nurse engagement benchmarking. This survey category must include a minimum of two pre-approved questions that reference nursing administration or the CNO.

Magnet® category
A dimension or subscale of registered nurse satisfaction/ registered nurse engagement or patient experience surveys identified by the Magnet Recognition Program and approved for Magnet reporting purposes.

Nurse Practice Act
"A statute enacted by the legislature of each of the states. . . . The act delineates the legal scope of the practice of nursing within the geographic boundaries of the jurisdiction. The purpose of the act is to protect the public" (Mosby, 2017).

nurse-sensitive clinical quality indicators (NSIs)
Indicators that are sensitive to the input of nursing care, reflecting structure, process, and outcomes (National Quality Forum, 2004). Measures that "reflect the quality of care given to patients by nurses" (American Nurses Association, 2016, p. 14). "Nurse-sensitive indicators (NSIs) articulate the value of nursing's contributions by measuring elements of patient care and patient outcomes that are directly affected by nursing practice. The identification and measurement of NSIs is critical in describing the contributions and value of registered nurses (RNs) in ambulatory care settings" (American Academy of Ambulatory Care Nursing, n.d.).

nursing practice
"Nursing encompasses autonomous and collaborative care of individuals of all ages, families, groups and communities, sick or well, and in all settings. Nursing includes the promotion of health, prevention of illness, and the care of ill, disabled, and dying people. Advocacy, promotion of a safe environment, research, participation in shaping health policy and in patient and health systems management, and education are also key nursing roles" (Bartz, 2010).

operational need
For Magnet purposes, an operational need is an identified gap that inhibits the ability of nurses to work in an efficient and effective manner (e.g., equipment, supplies, or time) to perform their jobs.

outperformance
For Magnet purposes, outperformance is achieved when the majority of selected categories/measures on the majority of units are better than the benchmarked mean, median, or other measure of central tendency provided by the organization's national benchmarking vendor.

patient experience
"The sum of all interactions, shaped by an organization's culture, that influence patient perceptions across the continuum of care" (The Beryl Institute, n.d.). For Magnet purposes, to measure patient experience performance is the act of gathering patient feedback surveys of quality care and comparing to national performance benchmarks to determine outperformance for improvement opportunities.

patient population
"Refers to the demographics and other particulars of a population being serviced—for example, a population's ethnicity, socioeconomic status, or population density" (Bowen, 2020).

peer feedback
An objective process of giving and receiving deliberate input to identify areas of strength and opportunities for improvement for a nurse peer. Professional nurse peers may include registered nurses with similar roles and education, clinical expertise, and level of licensure.

performance review

"A formal assessment in which a manager evaluates an employee's work performance, identifies strengths and weaknesses, offers feedback, and sets goals for future performance. Performance reviews are also called performance appraisals or performance evaluations" (Bamboo HR, n.d.).

professional development

"The activities, such as continuing education, advanced work practice, professional association involvement, teaching, and volunteer work, that credentialed professionals engage in to receive credit for the purpose of maintaining continuing competence and renewing a credential" (Institute for Credentialing Excellence, 2020, p. 15). See also *nursing professional development*.

Additionally, one of seven optional Magnet® categories for registered nurse satisfaction/registered nurse engagement benchmarking. This survey category must include a minimum of two pre-approved questions that reference education and resources.

professional practice model

"It is a schematic description of a system, theory, or phenomenon that depicts how nurses practice, collaborate, communicate, and develop professionally to provide the highest-quality care for those served by the organization (e.g., patients, families, communities)" (Silverstein & Kowalski, 2017). Professional practice models illustrate "the alignment and integration of nursing practice with the mission, vision, and values that nursing has adopted" (American Nurses Credentialing Center, 2013).

pulse survey

For Magnet purposes, a pulse survey for registered nurse satisfaction/registered nurse engagement is a survey that is not the organization's comprehensive annual or bi-annual satisfaction/

engagement survey. Pulse surveys typically ask fewer questions, track targeted measures or survey items, may be used to sample smaller subsets of the RN population, and are administered intermittently. Pulse surveys provide organizations an opportunity to respond to employee feedback and track the progress of associated action plans.

quality improvement (QI)
"In health care, quality improvement (QI) is the framework we use to systematically improve the ways care is delivered to patients. Processes have characteristics that can be measured, analyzed, improved, and controlled. QI entails continuous efforts to achieve stable and predictable process results, that is, to reduce process variation and improve the outcomes of these processes both for patients and the health care organization and system" (AHRQ, 2013).

registered nurse (RN) engagement
The concept of nurse engagement is often used to describe nurses' commitment to and satisfaction with their jobs. Additional considerations include nurses' level of commitment to the organization that employs them, and their commitment to the nursing profession itself. Nurse engagement correlates directly with critical safety, quality, and patient experience outcomes (Dempsey & Reilly, 2016).

registered nurse (RN) satisfaction
For Magnet purposes, registered nurse satisfaction is "expressed by nurses working in . . . [healthcare] settings as determined by scaled responses to a uniform series of questions designed to elicit nursing staff attitudes toward specific aspects of their employment situation" (Pollard et al., 1996).

RN-to-RN teamwork and collaboration
One of seven optional Magnet categories for registered nurse satisfaction/ registered nurse engagement benchmarking. This

survey category must include a minimum of two pre-approved questions that specify registered nurses rather than the broader team.

safety strategy

For Magnet purposes, a high-level plan that is designed to help workers meet one or more workplace safety goals. The safety strategy may be developed by individual workplaces, whole companies, or governments.

scope of nursing practice

"The description of the *who, what, where, when, why,* and *how* of nursing practice that addresses the range of nursing practice activities common to all registered nurses. When considered in conjunction with the Standards of Professional Nursing Practice and the Code of Ethics for Nurses, comprehensively describes the competent level of nursing common to all registered nurses" (American Nurses Association, 2021).

service recovery

One of nine optional Magnet categories for patient experience.

"The process used to 'recover' dissatisfied or 'lost' members or patients by identifying and remedying the problem or making amends for a failure or perceived failure in customer or clinical service. . . . Service recovery is about restoring trust and confidence in the organization's ability to 'get it right'" (Agency for Healthcare Research and Quality, 2020).

shared decision-making

For Magnet purposes, a dynamic partnership between leadership, nurses and other healthcare professionals that promotes collaboration, facilitates deliberation and decision making, and fosters accountability for improving patient outcomes, quality and enhancing work life (adapted from Vanderbilt University Medical Center, n.d.).

vendor
For Magnet purposes, a vendor can be an organization that provides benchmarked data or, alternatively, is an externally managed healthcare database that follows industry best practices specific to benchmarking. The vendor provides a national or an equivalent international benchmark comparison of an organization's data against other comparable healthcare organizations for the purposes of monitoring performance and prioritizing improvement opportunities.

well-being
Professional well-being is a function of being satisfied with one's job, finding meaning in one's work, feeling engaged while at work, having a high-quality working life, and finding professional fulfillment in one's work (National Academies of Sciences, Engineering, and Medicine, 2019).

workplace safety
For Magnet purposes, may refer to, but not limited to, initiatives designed to prevent musculoskeletal injuries, needlestick and sharps injuries, exposure to hazardous materials, and violence in the workplace.

workplace violence
Workplace violence is the act or threat of violence, ranging from verbal abuse to physical assaults directed toward persons at work or on duty. The impact of workplace violence can range from psychological issues to physical injury, or even death (National Institute for Occupational Safety and Health, 2020).

References

Agency for Healthcare Research and Quality (AHRQ). (2013, May). Module 4. Approaches to Quality Improvement. In *Practice Facilitation Handbook*. https://www.ahrq.gov/ncepcr/tools/pf-handbook/mod4.html

Agency for Healthcare Research and Quality. (2014, June). Chapter 2. What Is Care Coordination? In *Care Coordination Measures Atlas Update*. https://www.ahrq.gov/ncepcr/care/coordination/atlas/chapter2.html

Agency for Healthcare Research and Quality. (2018, February). *Ambulatory Care*. https://www.ahrq.gov/patient-safety/settings/ambulatory/tools.html

Agency for Healthcare Research and Quality. (2020, March). Strategy 6P: Service Recovery Programs. In *The CAHPS Ambulatory Care Improvement Guide: Practical Strategies for Improving Patient Experience* (section 6). https://www.ahrq.gov/cahps/quality-improvement/improvement-guide/6-strategies-for-improving/customer-service/strategy6p-service-recovery.html

Agency for Healthcare Research and Quality. (2020, November). *AHRQ Quality Indicator Tools for Data Analytics*. https://www.ahrq.gov/data/qualityindicators/index.html

American Academy of Ambulatory Care Nursing. (n.d.). *Nurse-Sensitive Indicators*. Retrieved April 9, 2021, from https://www.aaacn.org/practice-resources/ambulatory-care/nurse-sensitive-indicators

American Association of Colleges of Nursing. (2006). *AACN Position Statement on Nursing Research*. Washington, DC: Author. https://www.aacnnursing.org/News-Information/Position-Statements-White-Papers/Nursing-Research

The American College of Obstetricians and Gynecologists. (2018, January). *Cultural sensitivity and awareness in the delivery of health care: Committee on Health Care for Underserved Women Opinion, Number 729*. ACOG.org. https://www.acog.org/clinical/clinical-guidance/committee-opinion/articles/2018/01/importance-of-social-determinants-of-health-and-cultural-awareness-in-the-delivery-of-reproductive-health-care

American Hospital Association. (2021, January). *Fast Facts on US Hospitals, 2021*. Retrieved March 29, 2021, from https://www.aha.org/statistics/fast-facts-us-hospitals

American Nurses Association. (1979). *The study of credentialing in nursing: A new approach* (Vol. I, report of the committee). Kansas City, MO: Author.

American Nurses Association. (1996). *Nursing quality indicators: Definitions and implications*. Washington, DC. Author

American Nurses Association. (2015a). *Code of ethics for nurses with interpretive statements*. Silver Spring, MD: Author.

American Nurses Association. (2015b). *Nursing: Scope and standards of practice* (3rd ed.). Silver Spring, MD: Author.

American Nurses Association. (2016). *Nursing administration: Scope and standards of practice* (2nd ed.). Silver Spring, MD. Author.

American Nurses Association. (2021). *Nursing: Scope and standards of practice* (4th ed.). Silver Spring, MD: Author.

American Nurses Association and National Nursing Staff Development Organization. (2010). *Nursing professional development: Scope and standards of practice.* Silver Spring, MD: Author.

American Nurses Credentialing Center. (2008). *Application manual: Magnet Recognition Program.* 2008. Silver Spring, MD: Author.

American Nurses Credentialing Center. (2013). *2014 Magnet® application manual.* Silver Spring, MD: Author.

American Nurses Credentialing Center. (2015). *Primary accreditation provider application manual.* Silver Spring, MD: Author.

American Nurses Credentialing Center. (2020). *2020 Application Manual: Practice Transition Accreditation Program® (PTAP).* Silver Spring, MD: Author

Anthony, M. K. (2006). Professional Practice and Career Development. In D. L. Huber (Ed.), *Leadership and nursing care management* (3rd ed.; pp. 61–81). Philadelphia, PA: Saunders Elsevier.

Bamboo, H. R. (n.d.). *Performance review. An HR glossary for HR terms: Glossary of human resources management and employee benefit terms.* Retrieved April 11, 2021, from https://www.bamboohr.com/hr-glossary/performance-review/

Bartz, C. C. (2010). International council of nurses and person-centered care. *International Journal of Integrated Care, 10* (Sup), e010. https://doi.org/10.5334/ijic.480

Bass, B. M., & Riggio, R. E. (2006). *Transformational leadership* (2nd ed.). Mahwah, NJ: Lawrence Erlbaum Associates, Inc.

Benner, P., Tanner, C., & Chesla, C. (2009). *Expertise in nursing practice: Caring, clinical judgment, and ethics* (2nd ed). New York: Springer Publishing.

The Beryl Institute. (n.d.). *Patient Experience 101—Overview*. Retrieved April 11, 2021, from https://www.theberylinstitute.org/page/PX101

Bowen, C. (2020, February 12). *Patient Population*. Paubox. https://www.paubox.com/blog/patient-population

Burns, L. R., Bradley, E. H., & Weiner, B. L. (2012). *Shortell and Kaluzny's health care management: Organization, design, and behavior* (6th ed.). Clifton Park, NY: Delmar Cengage Learning.

Cain, C., & Haque, S. (2008). Organizational workflow and its impact on work quality. In R. G. Hughes (ed.), *Patient safety and quality: An evidence-based handbook for nurses* (AHRQ publication no. 08-0043) (ch. 31). Rockville, MD: Agency for Healthcare Research and Quality. Retrieved from https://archive.ahrq.gov/professionals/clinicians-providers/resources/nursing/resources/nurseshdbk/index.html

Curto, C., & Martin, D. (2020). The Magnet® site visit: Going virtual in response to COVID-19. *The Journal of Nursing Administration, 50*(11), 555–556.

D'amour, D., & Oandasan, I. (2005). Interprofessionality as the field of interprofessional practice and interprofessional education: An emerging concept. *Journal of interprofessional care, 19*(sup1), 8–20. https://doi.org/10.1080/13561820500081604

Darby, C., Valentine, N., De Silva, A., Murray, C. J., & World Health Organization. (2003). *World Health Organization (WHO): Strategy on measuring responsiveness*. https://apps.who.int/iris/handle/10665/68703

Dearholt, S. L., & Dang, D. (2012). *Johns Hopkins Nursing Evidence-Based Practice: Models and Guidelines* (2nd ed). Indianapolis, US: Sigma Theta Tau International.

Dempsey, C., & Reilly, B. (2016). Nurse engagement: What are the contributing factors for success? *OJIN: The Online Journal of Issues in Nursing, 21*(1), 2.

DePoy, E., & Gitlin, L. (2016). *Introduction to research: Understanding and applying multiple strategies* (5th ed.). St. Louis, MO: Elsevier.

Donabedian, A. (2003). *An introduction to quality assurance in health care.* New York: Oxford University Press.

Eggenberger, T., Sherman, R. O., & Keller, K. (2014). Creating high-performance interprofessional teams. *Am Nurse Today*, *9*(11), 12–14.

Epstein, R. M., & Hundert, E. M. (2002). Defining and assessing professional competence. *JAMA, 287*(2), 226–235. https://doi.org/10.1001/jama.287.2.226

Farquharson, J. M. (2004). Liability of the Nurse Manager. In T. D. Aiken, *Legal, Ethical, and Political Issues in Nursing* (2nd ed.; pp. 311–336). Philadelphia, PA: F.A. Davis Company.

Frankel, A., Haraden, C., Federico, F., & Lenoci-Edwards, J. (2017). A framework for safe, reliable, and effective care. *White paper.* Cambridge, MA: Institute for Healthcare Improvement and Safe & Reliable Healthcare.

Friedman, J. P. (Ed.). (2012). *Barron's dictionary of business and economic terms* (5th ed.) Hauppauge, NY: Barron's Educational Series, Inc.

Gardner, D. B. (2005). Ten lessons in collaboration. *Online Journal of Issues in Nursing*, *10*(1), 2.

Gourevitch, M. N. (2014). Population health and the academic medical center: The time is right. *Academic Medicine, 89*(4), 544–549.

Grawitch, M. J., & Ballard, D. W. (Eds.). (2016). *The psychologically healthy workplace: Building a win-win environment for organizations and employees.* American Psychological Association. https://doi.org/10.1037/14731-000

Griffith, J. R., & White, K. R. (2002). *The well-managed healthcare organization* (5th ed). Chicago: Health Administration Press.

Grossman, S. C., & Valiga, T. M. (2005). *The new leadership challenge: Creating the future of nursing* (2nd ed). Philadelphia: F.A. Davis Co.

Helmreich, R. L. (1998). Error management as organisational strategy. In *Proceedings of the IATA Human Factors Seminar* (pp. 1–7). Bangkok, Thailand, April 20–22, 1998.

Indeed. (2020, December 27). *Q&A: What is a professional organization?*. Indeed Career Guide. https://www.indeed.com/career-advice/career-development/what-is-a-professional-organization

Institute for Credentialing Excellence. (2020). *Basic guide to credentialing terminology* (2nd ed). Institute for Credentialing Excellence. https://www.credentialingexcellence.org/

Institute of Medicine. (2000). *To err is human: Building a safety health system.* (Kohn, L. T., Corrigan, J. M., & Donaldson, M. S., Eds.). National Academies Press (US). https://doi.org/10.17226/9728

Institute of Medicine. (2001a). *Crossing the quality chasm: A new health system for the 21st century.* The National Academies Press (US). https://doi.org/10.17226/10027

Institute of Medicine. (2001b). *Envisioning the national health care quality report*. National Academy Press. https://doi.org/10.17226/10073

Institute of Medicine. (2004). *Patient safety: Achieving a new standard for care*. (Aspden, P., Corrigan, J. M., Wolcott, J., & Erickson, S. M., Eds.). National Academies Press (US). https://doi.org/10.17226/10863

Institute of Medicine. (2011). *The future of nursing: Leading change, advancing health*. National Academies Press (US).

The Joint Commission. (2017). Patient Safety Systems (PS). In *Comprehensive accreditation manual for hospitals* (pp. PS1-PS50). Oak Brook, IL: Joint Commission Resources. Retrieved from https://www.jointcommission.org/patient_safety_systems_chapter_for_the_hospital_program

Kaya, N., Turan, N., & Aydin, G. O. (2015). A concept analysis of innovation in nursing. *Procedia—Social and Behavioral Sciences, 195*, 1674–1678.

Kindig, D., & Stoddart, G. (2003). What Is Population Health? *American Journal of Public Health, 93*, 380–383.

Lake, E. T. (2002). Development of the practice environment scale of the nursing work index. *Research in Nursing & Health, 25*(3), 176–188.

Laughlin, C. B., & Witwer, S. G. (Eds.). (2019). *Core curriculum for ambulatory care nursing* (4th ed.). Pitman, NJ: American Academy of Ambulatory Care Nursing.

Magnet hospitals. Attraction and retention of professional nurses. Task Force on Nursing Practice in Hospitals. American Academy of Nursing. (1983). *American Nurses Association Publications, G-160*, i–xiv, 1–135.

Malloch, K., & Porter-O'Grady, T. (2010). *Introduction to evidence-based practice in nursing and health care*. Burlington, Massachusetts: Jones and Bartlett Learning.

Merriam-Webster. (n.d.). *Merriam-Webster.com dictionary*. Retrieved March 29, 2021, from https://www.merriam-webster.com/dictionary

Mosby. (2017). *Mosby's dictionary of medicine, nursing and health professions* (10th ed.). Cambridge, MA: Elsevier.

National Academies of Sciences, Engineering, and Medicine. (2019). *Taking action against clinician burnout: A systems approach to professional well-being*. Washington, DC: National Academies Press.

National Advisory Council on Nurse Education and Practice. (2013). *Achieving health equity through nursing workforce diversity*. https://www.hrsa.gov/sites/default/files/hrsa/advisory-committees/nursing/reports/2013-eleventhreport.pdf

National Institute for Occupational Safety and Health. (2020, September 22). *Occupational Violence*. https://www.cdc.gov/niosh/topics/violence/default.html

National Prevention Information Network. (2020, October 21). *Cultural competence in health and human services*. https://npin.cdc.gov/pages/cultural-competence

National Quality Forum. (2004). *National voluntary consensus standards for nursing-sensitive care: An initial performance measure set*. Washington, DC: National Quality Forum.

NEJM Catalyst. (2017). What is patient-centered care? *NEJM Catalyst Innovations in Care Delivery*, *3*(1). https://catalyst.nejm.org/doi/full/10.1056/CAT.17.0559

Polit, D. (2010). *Statistics and Data Analysis for Nursing Research* (2nd ed.). Saratoga Springs, NY: Pearson.

Polit, D. F., & Beck, C. T. (2017). *Nursing research: Generating and assessing evidence for nursing practice* (10th ed.). Philadelphia: Wolters Kluwer Health.

Pollard, P. B., Andres, N. K., & Dobson, A. (1996). *Nursing quality indicators: Definitions and implications.* American Nurses Association.

Shortell, S. M., & Kaluzny, A. D. (2006). *Health care management: Organization design and behavior* (5th ed.). Clifton Park, NY: Thomson Delmar Learning.

Silverstein, W., & Kowalski, M. O. (2017). Adapting a professional practice model. *American Nurse Today, 12*(9), 78–83. https://www.myditialpublication.com/publication/?m=41491&i=435651&p=84&ver=html5

Titzer, J. L., & Shirey, M. R. (2013). Nurse manager succession planning: A concept analysis. *Nursing Forum, 48* (33), 155–164.

Vanderbilt University Medical Center. (n.d.). *Shared governance.* Retrieved April 11, 2021, from https://www.vumc.org/shared-governance/welcome

von Eiff, W. (2015). International benchmarking and best practice management: In search of health care and hospital excellence. *International Best Practices in Health Care Management,* 17, 223–252. https://doi.org/10.1108/S1474-823120140000017014

Weston, M. (2010). Strategies for Enhancing Autonomy and Control Over Nursing Practice. *Online Journal of Issues in Nursing, 15*(1). https://doi.org/10.3912/OJIN.Vol15No01Man02

Witmer, A., Seifer, S. D., Finocchio, L., Leslie, J., & O'Neil, E. H. (1995). Community health workers: Integral members of the health care work force. *American Journal of Public Health, 85*(8), Pt 1: 1055–1058.

World Health Organization. (2010). *Framework for action on interprofessional education and collaborative practice.* Geneva, Switzerland: Author. http://www.who.int/hrh/resources/framework_action/en/

World Health Organization. (2016, August 20). *Health promotion.* https://www.who.int/news-room/q-a-detail/health-promotion